Emotional Healing and Self-Esteem

Inner-life Skills of Relaxation, Visualisation and Meditation for Children and Adolescents

Mark Pearson

Jessica Kingsley Publishers
London and New York

The right of Mark Pearson to be identified as author of this work has been asserted by him in accordance with the Copyright, Designs and Patents Act 1988.

First published in Australia in 1998
by the Australian Council for Educational Research Ltd
19 Propect Hill Road, Camberwell, Melbourne, Victoria 3124, Australia

First published in the United Kingdom in 2004
by Jessica Kingsley Publishers Ltd
116 Pentonville Road
London N1 9JB, England
and
29 West 35th Street, 10th fl.
New York, NY 10001-2299, USA

www.jkp.com

Copyright © Australian Council for Educational Research 1998
This edition copyright © Australian Council for Educational Research 2004

Library of Congress Cataloging in Publication Data

A CIP catalog record for this book is available from the Library of Congress

British Library Cataloguing in Publication Data

A CIP catalogue record for this book is available from the British Library

ISBN 1 84310 224 2

Printed and Bound in Great Britain by
Athenaeum Press, Gateshead, Tyne and Wear

Acknowledgements

A special thanks to the seven contributors who shared ideas and exercises. To my partner, Helen Wilson, for careful editing and helpful suggestions. To Rosemary Pearson for editorial suggestions. To Ahrara Carisbrooke, who was instrumental in my personal growth and in the creation of the Emotional Release training courses. To Patricia Nolan, co-author on previous books, for encouraging feedback, and regular support through sharing case stories.

Using this book

Presenters should always refer to Chapter Three, 'A Practical Guide for Presenters' before embarking on the exercises.

The ideal way to prepare to use this work is for presenters to gather with a few friends or colleagues and explore the exercises together. The exchange of insights, interpretations, results and difficulties offers the best opportunity of expanded understanding. This provides more clarity on how to introduce the inner-life skills and program their progression for particular groups.

A few exercises have been adapted from material in *Emotional Release for Children* by Mark Pearson and Patricia Nolan (ACER 1995).

The author

Mark Pearson has worked as a primary school teacher in western Sydney. He has also run a remedial reading clinic and worked briefly with handicapped children. He is experienced with many types of meditation, and has worked as a meditation and relaxation instructor. He has been a trainer in ERC for over twelve years. He developed and directed training courses and personal development workshops at The Portiuncula Centre, Toowoomba for eight years. He currently conducts courses for ACER in Melbourne and, with partner, Helen Wilson, for *Turnaround Personal and Professional Development Programs* in Brisbane, Sydney and Melbourne, and around Queensland. He also travels around Australia presenting inservice programs for various agencies and government departments. Mark is currently completing further studies in Transpersonal Psychology with Stanslav Grof.

He is the author of the first Australian book on Transpersonal Breathwork: *From Healing to Awakening* (1991) and has co-authored *Emotional First-Aid for Children* (1991) and *Emotional Release for Children* (1995). His book *The Healing Journey* (1997) outlines the frameworks and modalities of ERC for adults.

Contributors

Dorothy Bottrell
Mary Martin
Elysha Neylan
Patricia Nolan
Paul Perfrement
Pat Quinn
Margaret Thomson

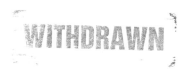
WITHDRAWN

Contents

Preface   **vii**
Introduction   **viii**

1 A new view of the landscape   **1**

Introducing inner-life skills   2
Code of respect   8

2 Acknowledging the silent ground   **9**

Using inner-life skills for personal development   10
Types of inner-life exercises   11
Basic principles   13
The place of emotional release work   15
Inner-life skills in school programs   16
Difficulties with quiet inner focus   18

3 A practical guide for presenters   **19**

Begin with your personal practice   20
Planning inner-life skills work   25
Recommended age ranges for exercises   27
Adapting exercises for different age groups   27
Practicalities for presenters   28
The value of integration   29
Group work   32

4 Feeling the warmth of the sun   **36**

Overview of methods   37
Self-awareness   48
Relaxation   53

5 Practising freedom, grace and beauty   **61**

Emotional and physical release as preparation   62
Slow-motion movement   70
Walking meditations   75

Contents

6 Journey to the centre of the Earth   **80**
   Quiet meditations   81
   Some basic stages   84
   Evoking the witness state   86
   Earthing exercises   90

7 Cultivating creative seeds   **98**
   A language for the inner world   99
   Visualisation   100

8 Reclaiming a lost world   **116**
   Focus on self-esteem: developing hope and inner strength   117

9 Attending to each moment of life   **130**
   Caring for your inner life   131
   The link between meditation and daily life   133

10 Building bridges through play   **138**
   Improving family and group communication   139
   General activities and exercises   140
   Personal development for parents   146

Appendix 1: Gestalt role-play question sheet   **150**
Appendix 2: Some cross-cultural sources   **151**
Appendix 3: Music   **154**
Appendix 4: Four Element Sheet   **156**
Resources   **157**
   Follow-up, support and on-going spiritual direction   158

Glossary   **159**
Index of exercises   **164**
General index   **166**

Preface

This book is partly a response to those parents, teachers and counsellors who have enthusiastically taken up the challenge of bringing elements of Emotional Release Counselling (ERC) into their daily contact with children, and have asked for more. It is also an expression of the energy, creativity and commitment of the members of the Australian Emotional Release Counsellors Association who have contributed to much of this material.

While working with teachers, counsellors, pastoral care workers and parents in ERC training courses around Australia I have been constantly impressed by the readiness for and interest in personal development in professional settings. The majority of those who come to courses and workshops express a dual interest in professional and personal development, and place the emphasis on their personal growth. 'I know that whatever I get from this for myself will really help the children I work with. So, I'm here for myself' they often say.

It is as if to become effectively altruistic we first need to understand and take care of ourselves. Self-awareness is the first step in caring for ourselves. Personal development is the ongoing work of self-awareness, emotional healing and the expression of new creativity. The exercises in this book are designed to meet this growing hunger for a deeper dimension in the inner life.

Many have found that as their own efforts towards self-development have come alive there has been a corresponding interest in self-discovery expressed by the children and adolescents they work with. There is then a need for more resources, more direction and more creativity. This book aims to support that creativity, and possibly lead you to its source.

Teaching children and adolescents inner-life skills for personal development is a major step in caring for the growth of their personality. These exercises and meditations will enable them to deal more skilfully with the emotional and psychological challenges of living in the world today.

The ideas and exercises here are drawn from several traditions as well as from the personal experiences of the contributors, who are all experienced and qualified in the areas of education, counselling or spiritual direction. The ideas and exercises have the common aim of supporting interest in self-knowledge and personal growth. No one approach has been the source. It has been our experience that a creative or spiritual component exists in all children and adolescents and that—given nourishing conditions—it emerges naturally from within.

Many of us feel that, in the light of the emotional conflicts, agitation and general lack of direction of the youth in our care, approaches that may have previously been considered luxuries are now essential for personal and academic growth.

Mark Pearson
Brisbane

Introduction

Our book, *Emotional Release for Children*, introduced the methods of ERC. It was warmly welcomed by counsellors, psychologists, child-care workers, educators and parents. It was intended to support deep emotional healing in children and adolescents through the release of blocked feelings and clear 'unfinished business' from the past. *Emotional Release* focused on the emotional release processes that can tap into the unconscious and bring profound positive changes in a client's psychology.

ERC has continued to become more widely studied and applied around Australia. It is now regulated by professional ERC associations and is the subject of several academic research projects.

This new book focuses on the inner-life skills component of ERC. These are intrapersonal skills that could be available to all children and adolescents as part of their basic education. Inner-life skills allow greater self-understanding, self-awareness, self-expression and self-help in the area of the inner world. This leads to a more balanced emotional outlook, a sense of self-worth and an improved ability to focus on learning tasks and developing positive relationships. The intent behind the book is to make these valuable methods more widely available.

Inner-life skills are often taught—directly and indirectly—by counsellors, and there is a rapidly growing interest from classroom teachers to include them in the school curriculum. The exercises in this book are suitable for personal development work in the classroom, during youth retreats, for families to play with, and for spiritual directors to implement as part of religious education. The exercises support emotional healing and lead to enhanced self-esteem.

CHAPTER ONE

A new view of the landscape

These forms of knowledge (the intrapersonal and the interpersonal intelligences) are of tremendous importance in many, if not all, societies in the world—forms that have, however, tended to be ignored or minimised by nearly all students of cognition.

Howard Gardner, *Frames of Mind*

Introducing inner-life skills

An 8-year-old girl reported after a visualisation exercise: 'In the middle of my island was a hut. This was the home of the unicorn. The unicorn was very brave. When I pretended to be the unicorn I felt brave too. Now when my brother comes into my room to annoy me I tell him to get out, and I pretend to be the unicorn again'.

The young girl now had a new way to access a brave part of herself. She reported that sometimes her older brother did do what she asked. This was a big change. For her, the image of the unicorn—along with the dramatic unicorn poster her mother bought for her as a reminder—allowed her to shift from victim mode. Having the imagery, the language and the experience of feeling brave gave her new self-esteem and helped her create the outcome she really wanted.

There is a wide range of sources for this approach to personal development. ERC, as developed in Australia since 1987, is based on the fact that our imagination and motivation have their source in the unconscious. This inner world has a major role to play in the emotional healing and self-esteem development of the individual.

There are three main strands of ERC:

• emotional release work—usually the domain of counsellors (see *Emotional Release for Children*)

• inner-life skills—the domain of teachers, counsellors and parents

• family communication games (see Chapter 10, pages 139 to 146).

These three strands can be used together to provide a child with the best possible support for emotional healing and self-esteem development.

The main inner-life skills explored in this book are relaxation, visualisation, meditation and active imagination. They support the development of what Harvard education writer and intelligence analyst Howard Gardner calls the intrapersonal intelligence (Gardner, 1984). They also make use of a range of activities that involve the child's mind, body, feelings and spiritual self.

Inner-life skills help children recognise their feelings and 'listen' to their inner world. These skills include becoming aware of imagery offered by the individual imagination. They help children express on the outside what is happening inside. There are seven main categories of inner-life skills that support emotional healing and personal development. They are:

1 self-awareness and self-knowledge includes:

2 learning to focus on the body

3 becoming more aware of the emotions

4 increasing awareness of beliefs about self, both positive and negative

5 increasing awareness of energy—flow and stasis

6 using relaxation, meditation, imagery, including symbol work.

7 understanding motivation and direction in life

1 Self-awareness and self-knowledge includes:
   - learning to focus on the body
   - becoming more aware of the emotions
   - increasing awareness of beliefs about self, both positive and negative
   - increasing awareness of energy—flow and stasis
   - using relaxation, meditation, imagery, including symbol work.

2 Understanding the unconscious includes:
   - dreamwork, working with fantasies
   - using guided reflection to review behaviour and beliefs
   - developing personal mythology from the imagination
   - awareness and reviewing of influence of cultural mythology
   - finding inner wisdom—intuition, inner guidance
   - acknowledging rites of passage.

3 Self-expression and communication includes using:
   - symbols as a source of creativity and self-understanding
   - line and colour
   - the written word
   - the spoken word
   - the body as a means of expression.

4 Managed emotional and physical release can take place:
   - solo
   - in pairs
   - in groups.

5 Relating to others includes:
   - recognising dynamics of group/classroom/family
   - dealing with negative reactions—projections
   - dealing with attractions
   - visualising and considering others' needs.

6 Supporting others includes:
   - practising active listening—partner work

- developing group awareness
- exchanging massage.

7 Understanding self-direction and motivation includes:
  - learning self-evaluation
  - working with visualisation
  - reflecting
  - finding inner wisdom
  - using energy creatively
  - identifying hopes and directions for the future.

For decades analysts, therapists, counsellors and spiritual directors have used the symbols of our dreams, fantasies and imagination to encourage emotional health and spiritual growth. They have found that there is a logic in the way imagination chooses and presents its images, even if this logic is not immediately clear to us. Inner-life skills offer many ways to connect with the inner world and listen for guidance. They are useful for children, adolescents and adults who are looking for a resource of creativity and self-confidence. These methods can often bypass the limits of the strictly rational way of thinking.

In some cultures there are general self-discovery methods woven into community life that are available to all. There are also esoteric methods reserved for pupils who have fully utilised the communal ways and gained a hunger for further development.

In our present age where instant gratification is the norm, there is often little willingness to put considerable time and effort into learning the steps to finding the inner world. However, any effort that can slow our incessant, automatic mind and calm jangled emotions can bring benefit. An awareness that there is a range of states of centredness, or calmness, may be the first step in activating the hunger for more. It may also activate an inbuilt interest in exploring the full potential of the inner world.

In communication with the author, some religious educators have reported turning more and more to the teaching of these inner-life skills. They find that the experiential work leads to a reverence for the self and others, as well as creating conditions for more subtle experience beyond the ordinary rational level of awareness.

There can be no doubt about the present need for more awareness, more sensitivity and more knowledge about our outer world. The only place this sensitivity can come from is the inner world.

This book presumes that parents, teachers, counsellors and youth workers will be willing to try out the exercises, perhaps with a group of colleagues or via an inservice course, before presenting them to children or adolescents. Inner-life skills exercises and personal development techniques, such as meditation, must at least be trial-run by presenters, if not thoroughly explored.

Emotional healing and self-esteem development

A 14-year-old girl, working on the last day of a three-day personal development retreat in New Zealand, found in her visualisation not a lovely animal nor a beautiful symbol, but a three-storey concrete car park! In the role-play stage of the exercise she 'became' the car park. It was empty, old, tired and beginning to crumble. Because her car park was on a small island it was not needed. As she played out the crumbling of the concrete pillars tears came to her eyes. 'I haven't been able to cry since I was a child,' she said. 'I was so sad yesterday in that group exercise, but a little voice inside said "stay strong!" I'm tired of being the strong one.' She quietly allowed her tears to flow and soon explained how onerous her load of chores—as the eldest of six—was at home. When she looked again at the car park, it had, in her mind's eye, changed to a playing field!

The imagery that comes from within the psyche during visualisation exercises always has relevance for a child's healing and growth. Sometimes it leads to direct feelings of empowerment and self-esteem. Sometimes it shows what feelings need to be dealt with or what issues are standing in the way of being fully alive. Inner-life skills programs should always use the self-discovery approach. There should be caution about presenters interpreting symbols or imagery that arise from the exercises.

These inner-life skills exercises are ideal for classroom use and many can relate directly to school curriculum aims of developing 'the whole child'. They support counsellors in assisting children and adolescents to find self-worth and trust in their own psyche. This trust is a prerequisite for the deeper emotional release work that many children benefit from. The relaxation and meditation approaches presented here greatly assist integration of emotional release work.

Many of the exercises in this book work well as family communication games (see pages 139 to 146 for details). Two, three or four family members gather together when and where they will not be interrupted. They make an agreement that they will respect the dignity of each family member, that they will not interpret or tell each other what to do or think or feel. During family communication games it is important for all members to receive equal time to speak and share their experience.

The exercises always work best when presenters have experienced them and personally felt their value. In so doing you bring an enthusiasm that helps children break through a possible first embarrassment stage.

Inner focus in action

A school classroom is quiet, with gentle flowing music. Twenty-six 8- and 9-year-olds are sitting cross-legged with their eyes closed. A few wriggle a little, peek around and then settle again. The teacher is describing a simple walk along the beach on a beautiful day. The words are calming, relaxing and comforting. She leads them in their minds to a quiet end of the beach where no one else comes. In their visualisation they sit and watch the waves. It is definitely time out from maths and reading. The part of their attention that is usually struggling to learn is now relaxing. The agitation, pushing, complaining and distraction of the morning has passed. There is a definite feeling of calm in the air. The children who find it most difficult to be still are sitting beside the teacher and she gently assures them with a light touch on the head.

After 15 minutes she invites them to bring their awareness back into the room, to stretch and wriggle. They then go quietly to their desks and draw. Some draw the scene they saw in their mind. Some draw shapes and colours and lines that represent the calm feeling inside them. A few write some words about how it felt to be still and quiet. Some are humming quietly to themselves. There is an atmosphere of settled focus. A debriefing follows. Each child's contribution is respected and encouraged. The others listen attentively. Soon they glide into the next lesson, using the words from the week's spelling list in sentences that go with their inner experience. This is a true story.

Creating relaxation, clarity and emotional stability

Emotional healing work, visualisation and meditation are not limited techniques. They are not just contemplating or introspection—thinking about things. They are not just mentally concentrating or limiting the range of awareness, or requesting something from a source outside. These activities are connected with active imagination, the Jungian method of following the flow of images that arise within. It can bring a new energy and lead to insights and an inner connection.

These exercises are not designed to fulfil needs of the ego. The ego, in this context, is the part of our psyche that thinks it knows everything, that protects and cuts us off from emotional and kinesthetic knowledge. The ego is always interested in doing something which is difficult because then there is a challenge. If you can battle a difficulty your ego will feel fulfilled. Surrender—a major step in all types of meditation—means a big shift for the ego.

All the exercises in this book can support children in this expansion beyond the limits of the ego. The controlling aspects of the ego work through our set thought patterns, limited and negative beliefs about ourselves and our rigid bodies that are kept braced against both the outer and inner worlds.

Children who have not developed emotionally will find it difficult to surrender. They have to hold on to the image of who they are. With practice, however, the experience these exercises bring will help them develop and feel better about themselves. Focusing within through creative imagination and meditation is like being a witness—practising the art of detached observation. Some call it a choiceless awareness that helps us come into stillness, into a poised, neutral state and move our attention away from the inner chattering. For many this awareness of inner chatter and hidden emotions, which may drive the chattering, is painful. The time of this awareness is often a time when the ego may wish to stop further exploration and discovery. Many children may actually need to spend some time with ERC methods before they see meditation, relaxation and self-esteem work as worthwhile.

Along with this poised state there is some action: that of letting go tension, expectation, analysis, ego direction and, most importantly, letting go of a tendency to force. Forcing, striving for awareness, struggling for stillness: all these are contradictions in terms.

The state of focused creative imagination can be recognised by a sense of watchfulness. We begin with watching and connecting with body sensation, then feeling our mood and its gradual changes towards the positive. The thinking state needs to be watched, that is, the movement of revolving, automatic thoughts as they begin to slow, quieten *or* redouble their efforts to distract us. And under all this is the finer vibration of inner energy, the pulsing of lifeforce. All of this awareness depends on the balance between action and non-action, remaining with, or in, the moment.

All this may seem too complicated for children and adolescents, but they do quickly appreciate each little step that helps them feel more secure, confident, creative and happy. When they see that teachers or carers value these methods, interest is awakened.

It seems that a harmonious inner state is only touched on briefly by us in our busy lives. We have not been educated to give a high priority to seeking this balance. Self-awareness exercises that begin to show us our lack of inner balance are an essential step in strengthening our motivation to pursue personal development.

Many who have pursued these types of inner-life skills, and felt the advantages of physical relaxation, intellectual clarity and emotional stability, have expressed a strong wish to pass these experiences on. All around Australia educators and child-care workers are incorporating these valuable methods into their programs and interactions with children and adolescents. They are finding new areas of the curriculum that can be enhanced by using relaxation, visualisation, symbol work and meditation as a teaching tool. Together we can add a new dimension to education, a dimension needed to face the daily challenges in our hectic world.

Code of respect

It is important that you adopt an appropriate attitude when introducing inner-life skills to children and adolescents. You need to:

- Uphold children's dignity.

- Understand and respond to acting-out as a symptom of the drive towards release and wholeness. The symptom may need the right time, place and support to complete its action in a therapeutic setting.

- Honour children's timing for trusting and their willingness to participate in inner-life skills. Each psyche has its own timing and logical reasons for that timing.

- Recognise that children's resistance, apprehension, procrastination and defences against the presenter, the methods, or their own inner world have logical causes—even if these are not immediately apparent to either the child or the presenter.

- Understand that children's need to feel safe may temporarily limit the choice of exercises, depth of work or duration of exercises and cooperate with this.

- Remember that nothing in this work should add to a child's lack of self-esteem. Lack of readiness in children to proceed can be seen as a challenge for the presenter to find the approach that will create trust, *not* as an inadequacy in a child.

- Respect the spiritual autonomy of children. It should be assumed that children are spiritual beings who may not yet have language to express their inner worlds.

CHAPTER TWO

Acknowledging the silent ground

Quiet times in the classroom not only
benefit learning, but also serve to
acknowledge the silent ground from which
language and cognition emerge.

S. I. Shapiro, *Quiet in the Classroom*

Using inner-life skills for personal development

Self-study leads to self-awareness, and self-awareness leads to self-knowledge. Self-knowledge can lead to choice, change and self-responsibility. Learning, through working with inner-life skills, some of the subtleties of how the body and mind function supports maturity. Being reconnected with the body through quiet inner focus exercises helps children become more aware of the needs of their bodies and how to take better care of themselves. Self-responsibility is a key factor in personal development. Why should young people wait until middle age to begin? Being more connected to the inner life helps us find direction for our outer life. Knowing motivation, finding calmness and understanding how we work create a stable inner base from which to make decisions.

Many children and adults let their attention wander, directed by whatever is the loudest stimulus, ignoring inner resources of creativity. Many children display short attention spans at school. There are a range of emotional and environmental factors that contribute to this. The right guidance and inner-life skills work can lead to an increased attention span.

An increase in the ability to concentrate leads to intellectual clarity and an increased readiness to learn. The author and contributors to this book have seen, and received many reports on, academic improvement over time in children who practise some form of inward focus and emotional healing. A development in inward focus leads to a more harmonious functioning of the mind, body and feelings and a general feeling of well-being. A relaxed body is part of this well-being which in turn brings improved concentration. There is also growing evidence that relaxation contributes to physical health.

Emotional stability can be another benefit of regular inner-life skills work. Children who are severely emotionally disturbed may not be able to work with stillness and quiet at first and would probably benefit greatly from some ERC (see *Emotional Release For Children*). However, finding the quiet place within, knowing it is there and even being able to return to it at times, brings a sense of hope and stability.

Bonding and group cohesion are supported when the results of self-awareness efforts are discussed and inner experiences shared. Personal development is greatly enhanced through group work.

Increased general creativity is a regular benefit of inner-life skills development. This work is also experienced and described as 'recharging your batteries'. The energy found in this work often flows naturally into expression such as singing a song, completing homework in record time, making up a story or finding new solutions to problems in life. A teacher of Year 10 students reported that the girls in her class had begun to write their own visualisation meditations. The exercises have been a boost to creative writing and to the recognition and expression of the real needs of the students.

Some cross-cultural sources

As there is no one basic source, the work here represents a growing synthesis of the offerings of Western personal growth pioneers, Eastern traditional practices and the Christian tradition of spiritual direction. (For further details see page 151.)

These inner-life skills methods come from a wide variety of sources. There is an urgent need to bring experiences of peace, calmness, balance and well-being to emotionally disturbed and agitated children and adolescents. This need has driven many of us to adapt our own experiences of both traditional and contemporary methods.

The author and the contributors have drawn on the methods of many cultures in their own personal development. Some come from the fields of spiritual direction, but present no dogma. Some come from the field of psychological and emotional healing, although they do not imply illness. Much of this work has been drawn from Jungian, Gestalt, humanistic, transpersonal and sacred psychology. This adaption and experimentation continues.

Some of the contributors to this book have found that the inner-life skills can be used with very positive benefit with children from non-Western cultures. The individual unconscious will yield insights and images that are culturally relevant for them.

Types of inner-life exercises

In a program that aims to teach personal development skills there should usually be a progression of work from simple to complex, concrete to abstract, just as there would be in an academic curriculum.

We recommend beginning instruction with simple self-awareness and relaxation (see Chapter 4). This will awaken the intrinsic interest in self-discovery and clarify motivation for further work. Self-awareness means awareness of the physical sensations of the body—for example, heat, coldness, tension, discomfort; the emotional mood—for example, depressed, sad, happy; and the inclination of energies—for example, restlessness, excitement, a feeling of deadness. The relaxation work allows the crossover from outer focus to inner focus, from doing to simply 'being'.

Only use the relaxation methods if they appear to be creating a positive result on a child's activity level or emotional state. If children are very agitated, need to run or jump, or are expressing destructively because of anger, they may become more agitated if required to remain still. In this case it would be more beneficial to use the active meditations, especially the bioenergetics, to release agitation (see Chapter 5). When using active meditations, as with all approaches, remember to move through the steps of:

- introduction, brief rationale, and overview
- a lead-in, perhaps with a demonstration and/or warm-up
- the experience of the exercise
- an integrating activity, such as recording, drawing, writing
- a discussion allowing for feedback.

Active meditations may include some brief emotional release work or bioenergetics as a prelude. Some exercises use slow motion to aid internal focus and body awareness. Some use dance and some simple walking accompanied by a specific task of focused awareness within.

These types of exercises—some of which are developed from the Zen tradition—are ideal for those children and adolescents who cannot sit still. It should be noted that after about 13 or 14 years of age adolescents will not readily dance or move freely when instructed to in formal exercises, and while being observed by adults.

Quiet meditations (see Chapter 6) can bring the benefits of calmness, extension of attention span, a sense of peace and happiness as well as relaxation and well-being. Initially many children will not be able to sit still for a long time and for some a long time is 3 or 4 minutes! These children may need you to provide stories, visualisations, imagery or reminders. However, these efforts should never result in more stress or a sense of failure. You will need to work at expressing acceptance and encouraging self-acceptance in the students.

Quiet exercises are usually most effective early in the day. If they are used in the late afternoon some movement or release work may be required beforehand.

Symbol work (see Chapter 7) allows an extended or new language to emerge so that children can recognise and express more about their inner world. Dr Carl Gustav Jung considered symbols, for example, in dreams and fantasies, to be the language of the unconscious. Children's interest in personal development is greatly encouraged by visualisations that allow them to fully use their imagination, or find images that represent their emotions, moods, qualities, memories, sensations or energies. This symbol work can support the emergence of new creativity in artwork, drama, vocal expression and writing.

Avoid telling children your interpretation of their symbols. The discovery method is vital here. Children should be encouraged to ponder the meanings of their symbols. This allows for the integration of aspects of their inner world that cannot be simply understood by the rational mind.

A focus on self-esteem (see Chapter 8) offers exercises that are designed to develop a sense of hope and inner strength. These self-esteem exercises help children acknowledge inner qualities that may not have been previously recognised or encouraged. All children benefit from these exercises and they are particularly useful for the 13- to 15-year age group, where negative self-images seem to abound.

A discovery approach—often using the simple Gestalt role-play (see page 150) or self-discovery questions—allows more convincing growth in self-esteem than some of the purely cognitive approaches.

Basic principles

Inner focus is not complicated. It is agitated minds that create complication. The experience of meditation and quiet inner focus is rarely instantaneous; it requires practice to progress in self-awareness. Effective work comes from a level of consciousness broader than the ego, beyond the ordinary daily level of awareness. It requires a shift in consciousness usually resisted by the ego.

The body is the starting point for inner focus. It is the container of our psychic state. Body, mind and emotions are closely linked. Many of us have been brought up in our culture with unconscious negative attitudes to our body. Part of all true self-development work is the increasing of this kinesthetic sense of ourselves, both in stillness and in activity. Inward focus can lead to a more harmonious functioning of body, mind and feelings.

Relaxation is a necessary part of this work. Children respond to words like 'floppy', 'melting' and 'falling inside yourself'. Transformation of energy, attitudes and self-knowledge ultimately requires a relaxed body.

Attention can be thought of as the opposite of tension. The very act of attentiveness to self can lead to relaxation, even though it may at first take us through a recognition of previously unknown tension. Inner focus can reveal long-held tensions that have been unconscious, and allow them to subside.

Emotional healing work with children is based on the simple premise that to acknowledge and feel emotions and energy and to let them be expressed—with support at appropriate times—supports mental health. The same applies to inner focus. Unless the emotional state is acknowledged, creative work cannot proceed effectively.

Negative feelings and memories, even in the unconscious, are active and have an influence on how we make choices and live our lives. Bringing them to consciousness is the first step in disempowering them. Positive qualities, feelings and memories in the unconscious tend to be inactive, or overshadowed by the negative. Making the positive qualities conscious allows them to be expressed and take their rightful place as a background to character. Using the inner-life skills will help you and the children you work with transform the negative into positive.

Both children and adults have an inbuilt interest in self-awareness and self-discovery which seems to be stronger at particular times in our lives. For many, mid-adolescence is a time of growing focus on the inner world. Sometimes this interest can be covered over by disappointment with life. Personal development work allows this interest to emerge again, forming a natural motivation for further exploration. Your role as a presenter of inner-life skills is to find the conditions for yourself and for others you work with that activate and enhance this natural curiosity.

The body, mind and feelings work as a whole. What we don't let ourselves feel or express becomes stuck and causes muscular tension, or 'armouring' of the body, and negative or destructive thoughts in the mind. This can lead to disruptive or destructive acting-out. Before attempting ongoing inner focus work it is important to release some of this tension. Work with relaxation and surrender allows children to touch the tender, loving feelings underneath the tension, and experience themselves as treasure.

As a regular part of inner-life skills, presenters should work towards releasing old shallow or restricted breathing patterns. Children unconsciously reduce their breathing in order to reduce their feelings and to contain excitement. Into any program build in some gentle ways to help breath open again.

As a prelude to quiet inner work, it is ideal to free up restricted sounding and movement patterns. Children usually have things to say, sounds to make, that have been stopped in their expression in the past. The impulse to express is still there, but contained. If not contained, it may have become a source of problems. It is this restriction in the body that can make quiet inner focus uncomfortable. Freeing the body makes its energy available to enhance awareness. Sometimes the freed energy can help connect children to a fuller experience of their potential.

Those who wish to begin teaching this work should spend time developing trust with the children they are working with. You need to help children recognise defence mechanisms, their ways of avoiding turning within, hiding or covering what is felt, denying their interest in self-knowledge, projecting a tough exterior. This defence is normal and soon gives way if you are confident, honest and really know the value of what is being offered. It is vital to accept resistance, nervousness, giggling and even choices not to participate. Inner-life skills cannot be forced or regulated. Your attitude should be one of invitation, never insistence.

It is important to give children a brief overview of some of the concepts of personal development and inner focus before you begin working with them. There is a need to satisfy cognitive levels and support their motivation to try new approaches.

It is vital that you are comfortable with and enthusiastic about the range and depth of the exercises and the experiences these exercises offer. Children need to sense that you are part of a safe environment in which they can feel and express themselves. We recommend that you experience the exercises with colleagues before presenting them to children.

Be on guard against projecting your personal needs or interests onto those you work with. To avoid this you could participate in some group work, or experiential inservice work which involve both inner focus and growth and healing work. Discussing your program with colleagues and parents will help you to clarify its direction and lessen any possible projection onto the children.

Presenters are models so there is a need for you to be engaged in your own personal exploration with the exercises. Those being taught will always sense any gap between what is being practised and what is being 'preached', and this may block the depths of new creative possibilities.

The place of emotional release work

Many questions arise for presenters with an interest in exploring and teaching inner-life skills. Do the children need release from disturbing, unresolved emotions? Most children need two elements: quiet inner focus and emotional release. However, any attraction towards inner quiet has usually been swamped because of habits of being entertained and 'filled up' with outside distractions such as regular television-watching.

You may have tried inner focus in your own personal development and then had to face a new level of emotional issues. You may have cleared some emotional problems and now long for quiet integrative experiences. So, what is the relationship between emotional healing work and deep quiet? How do we become totally feeling—in order to release blockage—and practise remaining a witness to our inner world? Can we live a more meditative life during our day *and* transform our so-called negative feelings? Do we accept the 'higher' in us along with the 'lower'? Before trying to teach this work ponder these questions. Clarity about ideals is essential.

There can be a flow between emotional release work, inner focus and the effort to be more sensitive and alert in each day. Each of us is reaching up in our own way and, like a pyramid, needs a strong base to support the small apex of inner effort that aims towards the heights. If we neglect the base, the apex will fall or remain unstable. If we neglect the pointing in the direction of wholeness we find little meaning in the base. Humankind is considered in many traditions to be between two worlds—material and spiritual. Ultimate fulfilment might depend on attainment in both worlds.

Since we are always automatically attracted by outer life, we need a conscious effort to listen to the life inside. This inner life needs our consciousness for its growth. The benefits of beginning this conscious awareness of inner life in childhood would be obvious to every adult who has made a serious effort to be still and quiet.

All this presupposes a certain amount of health—wholeness—in our psyche. This health may depend on clearing the negative patterns imposed by birthing and early childhood emotional wounding. Deep organic memories of confinement in the womb, the struggle of the birth and the immediate post-natal treatment can set up a drive in the psyche towards the future—the present is never felt as satisfying.

Dr Stanislav Grof wrote (1985): 'Like the fetus who is trying to escape from the uncomfortable constriction into a more acceptable situation, such a person will always strive for something other than what the present circumstances offer'. He suggests that this frame of mind generates a philosophy of life that emphasises strength, competitiveness and self-assertion—not the qualities that would turn one towards the inner life! So personal emotional healing, sometimes going right back to the womb, would be a vital step in creating an inner attitude that can appreciate life, creativity, imagination.

Exercising the inner-life skills in a group situation can be a good preparation for living daily life more fully. Active or dynamic meditations and bioenergetic dance work, when entered into wholeheartedly, increase awareness so that body, mind and emotions can be integrated, preparing the way to maintain a broader awareness in daily life.

These exercises can also address the chaos, the suppression, the conditioning, everything we have carried that needs to be healed. They allow a rare chance to express anger, tenderness, grief and joy, without getting lost in any one feeling. We can then merge with the freed energy, instead of being separated, blocked and full of oppositions.

Organised, formal inner focus exercises are a valuable educational tool. The results are a gift. After the exercise pondering may continue on the new questions raised. Adolescents in particular benefit from this new questioning about how they—and the world—function.

Some of the resistances to turning within may come from the 'creature' side of you and those you work with. Is there a possibility of satisfying the creature and the divine in us—so that all parts are satisfied? We may have to satisfy purely human interests, for example, social interaction, going to the cinema, etc., before this ordinary level will support us in devoting more time to focus within. Likewise children will not welcome quiet, still, inner work when their energy needs to be expressed on the trampoline!

Inner-life skills in school programs

The place of inner-life skills training in school programs may seem clear in schools based on a spiritual tradition. However, all schools can include it in programs that contribute to personal development and finding new creativity for written and spoken expression, artwork, drama and dance.

Educational aims of developing 'the whole person' sometimes leave out the emotional and spiritual components, or limit them to the province of counselling and religious education. Self-awareness work and inner focus can be blended into most subject areas, and the skills called on do contribute to developing the whole child.

There is a link here with developing the multiple intelligences—as identified by Gardner—through inner-life skills programs. Gardner identified seven areas or types of intelligence and emphasised that a balanced education depended on all seven areas being activated and extended.

The inner-life skills call on all of these seven areas.

Inner-focus work:

• can be taught as a life skill for emotional well-being

• teaches stress management and relaxation skills

• can act as a pre-lesson focusing device

• contributes directly to personal development through self-discovery

- contributes to spiritual growth and the arousing of philosophical questions
- helps children tap into their imagination and the creativity of their unconscious, especially in artwork and creative writing.

A lesson plan built around inner-life skills could include a range of ways children learn. For example:

- the guided discovery approach

- kinesthetic learning

- didactic input—giving simple information and frameworks

- emotional awareness development

- imitation with the presenter modelling

- using language—discussion, hearing oneself (especially in the integration stages)

- review—such as comparison of results of inner experiences

- reflection—pondering why certain feelings are there

- repetition—attempting the same inner focus exercise within a lesson, day or term

- visualisation—creating images and communicating these, following images given by others

- summary—especially at the end of a period of work.

Since schools are often a major site of created stress it would be ideal if the skills to resolve this stress were also taught. The attention stress-management work is receiving is growing. Many secondary schools now teach relaxation and use breathing to encourage calmness before exams. Children and adolescents who are beginning to learn to let go of school-related stress can also become more expressive about its causes. This in turn can help educators reduce or deal more successfully with the stress-causing issues.

Presenters of inner-life skills should use the usual teaching skills of breaking down the tasks, or steps, to the simplest stages, and teach these progressively and gradually. For younger children the introduction of stillness should be done gradually. Imagery is very helpful here. For example, being a forest blown by a gale that then quietens, being as slow as a tortoise or being as still as a rock.

Addressing the embarrassment that some adolescents feel when these 'weird' things are introduced is essential. Presenters and adolescents need to be able to laugh at themselves, together. Resistance, once expressed, is greatly reduced. Resistance should be seen as natural at the start, acknowledged, discussed and certainly not fought against. Many presenters report that initial awkwardness quickly gives way to keen interest and creative contribution when they are prepared and have gained confidence through trying the work themselves.

Difficulties with quiet inner focus

Agitation is a major difficulty in the practice of quiet inner focus. Agitation can be the result of conscious emotional disturbance, a high level of physical energy that does not want to be still, or some emotional turbulence that is unconscious, such as disowned anger. Often when children are dealing with death or loss, an accident, moving house or one of the major stressors, they will not be able to participate. In the case of emotional disturbance the attention will be constantly directed away from the inner world in order to avoid feeling emotional pain.

The requirement, or the effort, to be still can highlight the inner turmoil, even making it appear that the inner focus exercise has caused it! Children who carry a high level of turmoil will usually resent inner focus work at first and react against it.

Tension that is held deep in the body can come to awareness during stillness. Emotional or physical holding that has not been noticed in the busyness of life, can be discovered during quiet times, and this is uncomfortable. Again this can be interpreted by a child as 'This work makes me feel bad'. You may need to be prepared to allow for some movement or release of the physical holding before, during or after the quiet work.

Avoid setting up expectations. The aims or possible outcomes of inner focus should always be given generally so that no specific outcome is expected. We are all different and we experience differently. The same exercise may be experienced quite differently at different times depending on mood, energy level, motivation, disowned emotion, interest, etc.

Connected with expectations is the negative role of our inner critic, the judging part of ourselves. If we hold negative beliefs about ourselves—as most of us, including many children, do to some extent—the inner work experiences could be interpreted as proving these beliefs. Support for children to drop the self-criticism is essential. You should never add to these self-doubts by highlighting inability to be still and quiet. It should always be introduced as a learning process, with steps, however small, being made each time.

Some children have seen parents meditating and, of course, only seen the outward appearance of it. It is important that children are supported to have a reverential attitude towards all forms of inner work. Parents should avoid meditating in a place or at a time where children might feel neglected, or that they are missing out. Growing up with negative attitudes, resentment, or the impression that they already know what it is about, can rob them of real discovery.

CHAPTER THREE

A practical guide for presenters

The core capacity at work here is access to one's own feeling life—one's range of affects or emotions: the capacity instantly to effect discriminations among these feelings and eventually, to label them, to enmesh them in symbolic codes, to draw upon them as a means of understanding and guiding one's behaviour.

Howard Gardner, *Frames of Mind*

Begin with your personal practice

Most of us who teach and work with children are concerned with the practical things that we *do*. However, it has been our experience that children seem to learn most from what we *are*.

There is little use in teaching inner-life skills if you are not at the same time interested in your own inner world and becoming more relaxed. Isn't becoming more peaceful one of your greatest needs? Isn't it important to clear your energy and come to more awareness of yourself?

Working with this effort at self-awareness provides a direct model. Children perceive your state at a deep feeling level. That is what they really learn! No words can alter what they perceive as your inner state, your flowing or stasis of energy, your held or free feelings. Above all children long for and need us to be centred. This state of emotional and psychological balance can support a deeper relationship with children and, of course, with colleagues and loved ones.

Using your own experience

What is meditation? What is inner focus? It is certainly a very personal experience. However, self-awareness is not always pleasant. It often presents more questions to us than it answers. Most teachers, counsellors and youth group leaders agree that they can pass on, or share best, what they have explored themselves. The excitement, the enthusiasm and the challenges of your own self-exploration, your own personal development, can be a great gift.

So to plan and present to others you need to give yourself some stillness, silence, time and space. Ideas and themes for developing inner focus will grow out of your own experience. You will be able to choose programs and exercises that resonate with your experience and understanding, and teach more effectively.

Children need the stillness to feel their agitation, to hear the conflicting parts of themselves. They need the outer stillness to allow them to step out of the busyness and to let go in the body. Don't adults need the same? You need some relative silence in order to take your attention within, instead of having it attracted out all the time. You need silence to support your effort to meet your energies and relax from the mind-controlled state. You need time to feel 'at home' in your body, to know your feelings and to allow replenishment. Would it be too revolutionary to create time out for your inner self, and then to include this practice in your normal educational and care-giving activities?

Self-exploration exercise for presenters

Preparing myself to teach inner focus

Ask someone to read these instructions slowly to you, or read them through first.

Part one

1 *Lie down on a carpeted floor with a cushion under your head and close your eyes.*
2 *Visualise yourself at home early this morning. Visualise all the things you were doing, organising. Visualise each step up until you began reading this.*
3 *Feel the part of you that was interested to read more about inner-life skills.*
4 *Retrace each step, each feeling of your day until now, as if mentally watching a home video.*
5 *Become aware of your state now.*

Part two

6 *Focus on your energy. Can you differentiate energy, thoughts and feelings? What does your energy feel like? Where is it?*
7 *Is there a feeling of being more 'at home' in your chest? Belly? Hands? Legs?*
8 *Work for a few minutes to drop thought, to drop your awareness down from your head to your body.*
9 *Allow your body to relax more.*
10 *Watch. Become a watcher who does not judge; one who simply observes what is. Become very interested in your inner world, the world of sensation, feeling, thought, energy.*
11 *Let your awareness come to your breathing. Let the breath relax.*
12 *Let your awareness keep dropping down with each breath, let it drop into the core of yourself.*
13 *Let go of anything you already know about meditation, or how it ought to be, and watch inside.*
14 *Reject nothing, include everything in your watching.*
15 *Don't waste energy on berating yourself about distraction. Learn about any obstacles to becoming quiet inside.*

Part three

As you approach a quiet state you will be ready to lead your students to this same quiet, attentive, inner space in themselves.

16 *When you are ready, write down any insights and any ideas you have now about taking care of yourself with inner focus. Record the obstacles you found and keep these in mind for your discussions with the children you are working with.*
17 *When you feel ready, continue reading this chapter.*

Most of the initial work, before inner focus is enjoyable, might be clearing the deep hurts which have caused a closing off from the inner life. This is preparation for being truly still and awake. Buddha recommended the removal of the five 'hindrances'—sensual passion, ill-will, sloth, worry and perplexity—from the mind before meditation. Centuries later we still seem to need to do the same thing.

What will encourage your personal effort with inner focus? I sometimes use the reward method: a special French pastry and cappuccino if I can stay with the inner exercise for the full time. A regular place can help so reserve a room, a quiet corner or a special place in the garden. The habit, or ritual, of using this place will help.

To support the inner practice you need conditions where you will not be disturbed. You can make use of times in the day when the energy is naturally supportive, for example shortly after sunrise when the energies naturally awaken, and sunset, when everything begins to withdraw, become still. Although many of us feel trapped by routines, they can help. If you use the same time each day for inner focus the unconscious and the body begin to be ready for it.

Ritual can help to begin the quietening. All traditions include rituals. Create your own to begin to still the mind, relax the body, and connect to your wish, your motivation. Incense, candles and diffuse light evoke inward turning. Sometimes soft, sensitive music, created with a spiritual intent, can help.

It is important to avoid fighting yourself. Many of us have been brought up to struggle, to go against our natural self. Struggle is often a deeply ingrained approach to any learning task. You don't need it with meditation work! Try not to fight the mind directly. You cannot hold back the tide of flowing thoughts, images, memories simply by an act of will. Instead, turn your attention to sensation of the body. Where your attention goes, so also goes your energy. When you pay attention to the body some of the excess thinking energy can flow down into the body and you will feel quieter.

Repeatedly drop your expectations. You will see that almost all the time you have subtle expectations. The ego level of your mind cannot know what should or could happen. Its expectations are limited, and they stand in the way of recognising exactly what is happening. Let it all be self-discovery work.

Regular work to release the locked energy and wake it up is needed in a culture that promotes sedentary careers. Most so-called primitive tribes had rituals that did this. Sacred texts tell us that to know the divine we must come into resonance with it. Movement, dance, bioenergetics or walking meditation, followed by quiet still work, will support this resonance.

Here are a few helpful ideas that support letting-go, the ego shift and allow a state of simply watching and witnessing during inner focus:

• Remind yourself why you are making the effort.

• Acknowledge resistance, owning that many parts of you have no interest in meditation and would prefer to go to the cinema, etc.

• Check that posture is balanced and naturally stable with the least possible tension.

- Close eyes or gently fix them in one direction, for example, on a candle.

- Do not force breath. It needs to become soft, even and relaxed.

- Acknowledge that surrender would be the ideal state to begin from but recognise that it is not yet fully possible.

Nothing in particular is supposed to happen. There is a part of us that loves a struggle and wants to win. Can we make an effort that wastes no energy on struggle, and be open to any outcome?

Expectations, originating from the mind, take you away from the moment and acknowledging how you are. Once awareness is attained you can relax from doing anything in particular. This awareness can expand so that you move through being occupied with the contents of consciousness—our emotions, thoughts, plans, memories, images, stories, body sensations—to *being* consciousness.

ERC methods clear negative emotion and chronic body tensions through expression and release. Bioenergetics, especially when done to rhythmic music can awaken our energy (see page 64). The body and mind can be harmonised through structured movement, for example, Tai Chi and yoga. We can also use free dance to awaken the body and redistribute excess 'nervous' energy. Inner chaos can be mirrored with cathartic methods: merging with chaos, expressing it so fully that harmony results.

Sounding and humming are used in many traditions to vibrate the inner energy system and recharge the brain. We know that the early Christians used mantra prayers and special songs to resonate with, and have a positive impact on, their body energy.

Having previously prepared yourself through active exercises, you can recognise some basic stages in quiet sitting work (see page 84). There is that initial sense of coming home, beginning to 'anchor' awareness in the body. This begins with focus on physical sensation—especially in the hara, the energy centre in the belly. With an active effort to pay attention, which includes watching the evolving receptivity, breath becomes more open. Patient persistence may lead you to a state that has been called the 'creative emptiness' where you will feel new energy flowing in. Subtle, positive feelings resulting from the new harmony in this finer state can emerge and you may sense some new creativity bubbling up inside.

Can there be danger in quiet inner focus?

The main difficulty that can arise from quiet sitting meditation both for children and ourselves is one of emotional and physical stress if the exercise has been forced. The exercises are supposed to reduce stress, but if a child or adult forces stillness and narrow concentration, with an attitude of needing achievement, this can actually increase stress. Also if exercises are used without regard to children's need for release of agitation or expression of impulses to move, there could be some acting-out when students are released from the class.

Some meditation methods in old Western traditions utilised body energy and allowed for quiet preparation of the mind. They were used in the context of a rigorous life of physical expression. For example, the Greek Orthodox Church had much ritual that involved bowing, prostrating, sitting and standing.

Methods that utilise long periods of sitting, such as Vipassana or ZaZen, should only be carried out under experienced direction, and not mixed with emotional release work. They were designed for people leading a strenuous physical life, and for those who cultivated a surrendered ego. Unsupervised, they could possibly lead to more stress.

Psychic phenomena which occasionally occur for some adult meditators—such as lights appearing, auditory phenomena—should be included in the awareness, but not given the focus, and most certainly not sought. Be wary of identification with states and experiences. Looking for results and pride in achievement are two ego states that are familiar but are not helpful. Once recognised they can be dropped.

In all traditions there are warnings about working only for personal gain, and about beginning from self-will. Inner work is often begun with a prayer dedicating the effort to the good of all. Do you seek something beyond your personal self in the meditation work? Can you make use of your efforts in the support of others?

Progress in quiet inner focus

The question of progress in inner work is often raised. Is there progress with meditation? How could it be recognised? How can you be sure that you are not compounding some mistake? A simple test can be to ask 'Am I becoming more peaceful? More satisfied? More accepting?'

There are signposts that inner focus is progressing in a healthy way. With practice you may come to:

- an inner silence that becomes more accessible and deeper *or* an increase in the ability to watch the chattering without judgment

- a deeper connection to the energy in the body and more frequent pleasant sensations of it buzzing, vibrating, tingling or expanding

- a stronger feeling of balance and connection to a sense of your centre

- more frequent moments of feeling 'at home' and attentive to the present moment

- pleasant body sensations that begin to attract wandering awareness back home

- much less inner reaction to others, more freedom

- more vital senses—the trees seem greener, the air crisper, the sounds clearer and more musical—although there may also be more sensitivity to abrasive sounds

- moments of 'waking up' in daily life, of becoming more self-aware while being engaged in daily life.

All this brings a feeling of delight and creativity. There is more self-awareness and confidence directing your life.

Planning inner-life skills work

Planning and presenting an exercise or a program of inner-life skills can be challenging and very rewarding. Following is some general advice aimed at enhancing the effectiveness of the work. It will also help you through possible early stages of resistance from the children.

- Know your reason for presenting the exercise and consider what children's reasons for opening to it would be.

- Begin with surrender, relaxation, letting go. Little real inner growth or healing takes place while the ordinary mind is in charge. Surrender—lying down, closing eyes, relaxing the muscles, dropping thoughts—is the state to aim for. The state of surrender allows the welcoming of subtle experiences that bring great positivity.

- Encourage an open posture of body. Be aware if there is hesitation to open, or if it feels uncomfortable. The open posture may challenge the usual defensive, protective attitude so do not insist on it.

- Make any resistance, fear or embarrassment conscious. Talking about it, expressing it, bringing it out into the light, reduces its power.

- Use suggestion to help relaxation. For example: *Feel your body softening. Feel your shoulders dropping the weight they have been carrying.*

- Inner focus could develop from the effort to turn attention to the body sensation. Perhaps begin by becoming aware of the weight of the body on the floor or cushion, the feel of clothing, the temperature on the skin, then moving inside to feel heat, pulse, vibration of energy, emotional flow.

- At first keep the attention moving in order to discourage children from losing concentration. They are using your will, your presence to begin with. Attention should move at a speed that allows inner contact to begin but keeps children attentive.

- Remind children to let go of distractions such as wandering thoughts, physical discomfort, the associations begun by sounds, plans to do the exercise better another day! Introduce acceptance of the idea of beginning over again.

- Remind children that the aim is practice, not achievement. Let go of expectations and waste no time on judgments.

25

- Encourage children to contact the emotional mood or inner attitude. Simply be aware of this, acknowledge it.

- Decide whether there will be a main area of focus such as the heart, the hands or the hara (belly). Have a reason for choosing this focus.

- Sometimes it can be helpful to give the mind something to do, for example, a mantra (a repeated word or sound), an order for focusing such as becoming aware of each limb in turn, an instruction that might include counting or a rhythm.

- Include an invitation to open to more than the ordinary self, something more conscious, higher, finer.

- Present exercises as questions, experiments, opportunities to learn more and not as definite formats with set outcomes. Remind children that they cannot go wrong, cannot make a mistake because whatever happens is material for self-knowledge, for new learning.

- When it is time to bring children's awareness back to the outer world, do it gently and slowly. Maybe suggest a gradual reconnection with the posture and weight of the body, to the breathing, to small body movements, for example, wriggling the toes or spreading the fingers before slowly opening the eyes. Invite them to stay connected within as they include the outer world. Encourage them to have a short experience of divided attention at this time—being connected both within and without.

- Integrate through drawing, writing, modelling, sharing with one other, before asking for group sharing. Sometimes quiet inner focus experience is profound and is best not talked about. Respect any need children have not to discuss their inner experience.

- Invite participants to compare their state before and after the exercise. Using a body outline drawing (see *Emotional Release For Children* page 64) to express the inner experience before and after the exercise is a way to help them evaluate what has happened.

Exercise for presenters

Questions to ponder when preparing exercises

1 *What do you hope to achieve for the group through the inner focus?*
2 *What is the main outcome you would like for individual children?*
3 *What is your own main obstacle to quiet awareness and stillness? For example, inner talk? Body tension?*
4 *What difficulties do you encounter in quiet inner work? How do you deal with these?*
5 *How can you help children deal with similar difficulties?*
6 *What is the children's energy, mood and attitude right now?*
7 *Is the timing right for quiet work?*
8 *Is movement or release work needed first?*
9 *Do you ever get to an experience of inner silence? How will your personal experience help you in presenting?*

Recommended age ranges for exercises

Many exercises give a minimum age and suggest that the exercise is suitable for all ages up to adults. Obviously there may have to be some changes in vocabulary for different ages, even if the structure and method of the exercises remains the same. Although a minimum age is suggested, in some cases children younger than this would be capable and willing to try the exercises. Changes in vocabulary may also have to be made to suit the cultural background of participants.

There will always be a variety of responses to the exercises in this book. It is quite normal for children who are trying the exercises for the first time to express some hesitancy. Those over the age of 10 may be more self-conscious—and therefore more cautious—than younger ones. The self-consciousness of those between about 10 and 17 years of age can be quite strong. This may mean that they take some time to become comfortable with inner-life skills, and will initially resist any exercise that involves physical expression, movement or self-revelation.

The types of preparation—cognitive input, setting, etc.—that are mentioned throughout the book are essential in introducing inner-life skills for the first time. This preparation may make the difference between acceptance and co-operation and low-key participation.

Most of the exercises have also been used with adults within our ERC training courses and they regularly report a positive experience and deep interest in the experiences evoked.

Adapting exercises for different age groups

The main differences you will find between the age groups you work with will be the time you spend on an exercise and the language used to introduce and structure it. Different age groups have different natural interests. If these are discovered and addressed the work will flow very successfully.

For example, children up to about 9 years will enjoy a focus on things connected with nature and fairy stories. Many 9- to 12-year-olds will respond well to adventure stories or elements of adventure in the exercises. They will be more able to identify and express feelings. Children over 12 may find problem-solving an interesting challenge. Remembering this can help you choose or create visualisations.

For younger children liberal use of imagery will be helpful. For example: *floppy like a puppy asleep in the sun, flowing like a silk scarf when you twirl, still as a rock in the desert.*

Practicalities for presenters

If working with a group it is ideal to have two presenters: one to keep contact with the whole group, one to attend to or encourage individuals if needed. The following can provide a checklist to improve your preparation and presentation.

• Always experience the exercises yourself before presenting them.

• Before presenting, review the exercise carefully. Is the language appropriate for the age group you are working with, and for their social and cultural backgrounds?

• Always repeat your instructions at least twice. Then look carefully to see if you have been understood. Do you need to rephrase the instruction?

• If using background music always check its suitability first. Turn it down as you give instructions. Rewind tapes, and have other options ready.

• Make it clear at each stage whether you want children's eyes to be open or closed, when you want them to look at you, relate to each other or stay focused within.

• Give a brief overview of the aim and sequence of the exercise before presenting it.

• If partner work is involved, ask children to choose partners before giving introductory instructions.

• If you sense resistance in children get them to talk about it and make it conscious before beginning the exercise. This decreases the resistance.

• Set up and order the work space before beginning—preferably before children come in. Check you have any materials needed.

• Always familiarise yourself with equipment before presenting. For example, it is amazing how often the volume control on the cassette player disappears when you are in the middle of an exercise!

• Be sensitive and flexible about time. Watch the attention span. Give time boundaries clearly and give time warnings when it is nearly time to stop an exercise, or a section of it.

• Talk to the children about the need for confidentiality in the discussions.

• Close curtains or blinds and dim lights so that children's eyes can relax in a gentle light. This also helps the focus be turned within as there is less connection to, and distraction from, the outside world.

• Make sure the work space is delineated. For example, cushions or chairs can set the boundary if working in a large hall. Order, tidiness and beautiful impressions are also important and help to make a space psychologically safe.

- Help the supporters during partner work by giving clear instructions and occasionally making eye contact with them to indicate 'all is well'. This is particularly important if the person they are supporting is feeling emotions.

- A simple way to evaluate the work after an exercise or a series of exercises, is to ask the children to write down some words or phrases which best describe their responses to the activities. The responses will give the facilitator confidence to proceed. Evaluation brings the intellect into a new relationship with experiential work and opens students to integrated understanding.

Note: Teachers should not be put off if stuck with rows of tables and chairs, grey walls and no blinds! It is certainly still possible to do good work. The teacher's and students' attitudes are much more significant in creating the right atmosphere. Children can be very flexible.

The value of integration

Most exercises in this book are completed with an integrative action:
- writing
- drawing
- dancing
- choosing a symbol
- proclaiming—making clear statements about self
- one-to-one, or group sharing of experiences
- celebration.

This kind of integration at the time of the exercise is ideal.

After working with a group a few times it is good to ask for feedback. Simple questions such as *'Do you think of the things you learn here in between times?'* Such questions can help a child begin to connect inner work and daily life.

Another simple method to support integration is to review completion drawings that have been collected together in a child's special book or folder. Reviewing these experiences and reading the summary words that accompany the drawings, or reports in their journal, can highlight the extent of children's experience and depth learning. Be clear before inviting journal writing if it is private or if you wish to read it.

A very important aspect of the process of integration is letting the new energy exist and be fully felt and expressed in and through the body. Dance and celebratory movement can help here.

Drawing

In exercises that use crayons to express inner images and states it is good to say: *'What colour is it? What colour feels right for that?'* This is a way of helping a child to look within more carefully. The intensity or faintness of the colour, its softness or hardness, firmness or tentativeness are all subtle expressions of the inner state of the child in that moment. It is not important for presenters to understand or be able to analyse children's drawings.

When imagination presents an image from the unconscious or new contact is made with an unfamiliar state it is good to record it. All too often the clarity of the experience can slip away. A drawing is a way to bring new learnings into life. It can be used as a basis for further discussion and exploration. Drawings are very useful in encouraging expression from inarticulate children. To draw when their connection to the energy of an exercise is still alive allows it to live in children. The energy can then be released, integrated or celebrated as needed.

Mandala symbolism

A mandala begins with a circle marked out on a blank page. We frequently invite children to do their completion drawing in a circle.

The circle can give a feeling of safety. Some Jungian researchers have found that it is of therapeutic value to draw inside a circle. Using a circle as a starting point for completion drawings is far more soothing and inviting—visually and emotionally—than a rectangle.

In discussion with children you might find that symbolically this circle can represent themselves now, or in the past, or it can represent their family, the world, their energy. What is placed inside and what is placed outside the circle can indicate their feelings about relationships and about boundaries.

Reviewing completion drawings and mandalas

After a series of inner-work exercises it is good for integration to review the drawings and mandalas. Remember the intention may be to draw something specific, but drawing also comes from the unconscious. There may be much in a drawing that was unintended on a conscious level by the child. So in review, study these mandalas from both levels. Invite children to look again and discuss what they intended to draw and anything they think that their inner world (unconscious) might have wanted to draw.

No interpretation by you is required. In fact it can stop children's exploration and self-discovery. This may require that you let go any training about the need to explain things to children, giving them insights or being the 'expert'.

Mandala review exercise

What do my mandalas say?

Age range: 12 years to adult.

Older children could work in pairs, younger ones with the presenter. Spread out drawings from a series of exercises so that all can be seen at once. You will need extra drawing paper.

1 *Look quietly at the drawings for a moment.*
2 *Which ones could be extended off the page, which ones want to grow more?* (Give out extra paper to allow this to happen.)
3 *Look at strong and weak colours and lines. What does this mean to you?*
4 *What themes seem to emerge? Check colours, shapes, moods, repeated symbols.*
5 *Is there some sense of progression in the drawings? For example, dark murky colours to happy bright colours or jagged chaotic lines to curved flowing lines?*
6 *What do the drawings say to you right now?*
7 *Are there any clear divisions? Splits? Changes?*
8 *What symbols have some special attraction for you?*
9 *Would it be helpful to use the Gestalt role-play questions to understand your mandala symbols more fully?* (See page 150).
10 *Write a short statement about your discoveries so far.*

Recording through journal writing

The idea of ongoing personal development can be emphasised with older children. Sometimes it is referred to as journeying. One of the methods which assist a sense of individual journey is the keeping of a journal. Children must have the right to keep their journals private. They should be able to choose what they show to others.

For younger children simply call it 'your special book'. Encourage them to write or draw a record of their work. It is a way for them to have a personal and private record of their inner world. Some like to use it as a diary. The actual writing can be a process of growth and change. Guiding questions for journal writing are often given at the end of the exercise or you can create questions or topics that are relevant to the moment.

Discussions

Group times to share experiences from the exercises enhance the integration and understanding of inner-life skills. Discussions have many purposes, and support children in finding clarity and practising expression.

They create a bonding with a group and allow you to assess the success of the program. Talking about inner work will usually ensure that the ordering and structuring functions of the mind come into play and this helps complete integration.

Purposes of group discussions for children
Group discussion for children:

• enhances integration of inner experience

• gives children the chance to hear themselves speak about their experiences which in turn helps to clarify them

• removes a sense of isolation that many children live with around their inner world

• allows children to proclaim something new about themselves, and to honour and confirm their inner discoveries

• gives the experience of uninterrupted attention from presenter and group

• creates a bond within the group that will support future work

• develops trust that will then allow further work in the future

• develop skills of expression.

Purposes of group discussions for presenters
Group discussion allows you to:

• gauge the effect of the exercises through hearing what is discussed as well as listening to the voice energy and watching the body language

• take time to give guidance for further work

• clarify any misunderstandings about the exercises or the conceptual frameworks

• check there is group cohesion.

Group work

Many presenters will be teaching inner-life skills to a group. The following notes are intended to support those new to presenting personal development work to groups.

Note: A group formed for inner work is most effective with about six to ten members. If it is necessary to work with a larger number create sub-groups that can easily form a bond and sense of group identity. Initially group work may be more effective if best friends are placed in different sub-groups.

The benefits of group work

- Ideally groups will provide sympathetic ongoing support where children can learn that it is okay to let their inner world show. The composition of the group should remain the same to help sustain trust and confidentiality. This allows children who have 'broken the ice' and dropped their defences to remain comfortable with the group.

- Some children may experience feelings of acceptance for the first time in a group. Acceptance from the outside helps self-acceptance.

- Group work supports the learning and practice of the skills of support.

- Leadership skills and confidence can develop from group work, especially when individuals have the chance to lead small sub-groups.

- When young people share inner world experiences they go through the risk of exposing themselves and very quickly form a close bond. Self-disclosure is the fastest way of creating a bond. It is also perhaps the riskiest activity and needs sensitive, aware support from presenters. It is important that self-disclosure is never demanded or forced by the group or presenter.

Structure of groups

- Work with at least two presenters. One can focus on the presentation to the whole group and stay tuned in to the general group energy and readiness. The other is free to move about and give individual encouragement as needed. Presenters should be clear about these roles.

- In a school setting where the group session is timetabled into a busy day it may run for forty minutes and allow the exploration and integration of only one exercise. In a retreat or workshop setting more time will be available, but the group will need clear beginnings and endings as new work is introduced.

- Frequent breaks are essential. A rhythm of gathering together, inner focus, sharing, integration, recording and relaxation, then a change of scene, pace or modality is advised, especially in workshop or retreat settings.

- Frequent breaks and unstructured times also allow for peer group discussion. This is very important for young people so that they can connect with each other at a deeper level. This sense of community can develop well in a retreat setting and encourage the ongoing benefits of increased social cohesion after the retreat time.

Problems for presenters

One of the most challenging situations for presenters working with a group of older children is the high level of resistance that can be shown by some participants. This can slow the rate of work for the whole group. Remember that resistance is often a sign of fear and there will be clear reasons for it even if they are not understood by the children in question.

Your challenge is to deal with this positively. Those that resist inner exploration and revealing of anything personal can actually mirror and even trigger-off your unacknowledged resistance. You will know this is what is happening if you are experiencing a *reaction* to these particular children.

When you have worked through your own hesitations and resistance these children no longer seem a problem to you. A creative new way emerges to support their real need at their level of readiness and alternative activities or new ways of structuring the work will emerge. These will enable those resisting to participate at some level. And they will be more willing without the added load of your irritation.

Those who resist are actually those who are most frightened. Remember that under their fooling around, under their disruption, is their fear. They may even need some private work to release the held-in emotional problems behind the fear, before being ready to try meditations.

Obviously resisters must not be forced in any way, or made to feel inadequate. Sometimes they are simply the ones who take longer to develop trust and 'break the ice'.

Note: It is almost impossible for presenters to act as authority figures and be responsible for children's behaviour to and from the workshop or group. Children and adolescents will rarely open up to an authority figure. This is why teachers and parents are often unable to help their own children as much as an outsider or someone who only has a support role, for example, grandparents, camp leaders, the school counsellor.

Exercise for 'breaking the ice'

Getting to know each other

Age range: 12 years to adult.

Use this exercise when beginning group work with older children. It is a simple way to ritualise first meetings and begin to 'break the ice'.

1 Set up the room with two concentric circles of chairs or cushions in pairs. The number of chairs or cushions should coincide with the number of children in the group.

2 Ask members of the group to choose a partner, then sit opposite each other. If they have not met before, they introduce themselves and make sure they know each other's names.

3 Read out the following list of questions, one at a time, for the children to talk about with each other.
   - *What things make you uncomfortable about this group work?*
   - *What do you like most about this group work?*
   - *What things really annoy you in your life at the moment?*
   - *What is your strongest or best quality?*
   - *How many brothers and sisters do you have? Where do you come in the family?*
   - *What things make you sad? What things make you happiest?*
   - *Is there anyone in your life you are afraid of?*
   - *How do you feel about being in this group right now?*

4 Before each question direct children to:
   - become still
   - close their eyes
   - take a full breath
   - feel what is going on inside themselves
   - give their inner self time before rushing to answer the questions.

5 When the children have had a moment of inner contact they leave their eyes closed as you read out the question. They wait and see what presents itself in their minds, then they ponder the question for a moment. When children are ready to talk they open their eyes and share.

6 After each sharing children sitting in the outer (or the inner) circle stand and move on to the next chair or cushion on their right.

7 Vary the number of questions to suit the time available and the interest level. If there is time, children can choose to meet someone from their own circle to share with as well.

8 Complete the exercise by asking children to return to the first person they partnered and discuss how they felt about the exercise.

CHAPTER FOUR

Feeling the warmth of the sun

... and I believe that this is the great thing to understand (that awareness per se—by and of itself—can be curative). Because with full awareness you become aware of this organismic self-regulation, you let the organism take over without interfering, without interrupting; we can rely on the wisdom of the organism.

Fritz Perls, *Gestalt therapy verbatim*

Overview of methods

To gain access to the creative side of imagination children need some relaxation. To focus their creativity requires some degree of self-awareness. The greater the degree of self-awareness and relaxation, the greater the possibility for accessing and directing creative energy in a positive way.

What makes an exercise a self-awareness exercise?

• The intent should be to learn, not achieve.

• The atmosphere should be one of relaxation and enjoyment.

• The attention should be directed within to assess:

– the state of the body

– the emotional response to the exercise

– the intellectual insights gained.

Some articulation of what has been observed can also be helpful and sometimes comparison, through group discussion, is valid to help participants know if their experience is unique, similar to others or the common response.

It is vital that children know that there is no right or wrong way to do the exercises. Unlike other academic subjects, it is purely the experience and insight gained that is important, not a specific outcome.

Each of the following methods can be explored as an experiment, ideally without time limits. Generally it is a good policy to do any actions slowly. Most of these methods are ideal for group work where children work in pairs.

Releasing body energy as a preparation for relaxation

These approaches are particularly useful for beginning work with disturbed children who are out of relationship with themselves and others as a result of emotional problems. Preparation for quiet and still work can be through:

• hand, foot or shoulder massage in pairs or trios

• bioenergetic games (see examples on pages 64–65)

• shaking and dancing

• running and sport

• time on the trampoline.

Breathing

Full and free breath can facilitate connection to the inner world. Focusing on the breath without any interference can bring more awareness of sensation and lead to a quieter state. This quieter, more peaceful state may begin to emerge after a few minutes of quiet focus on breath. It will be recognised by the sense of calmness that goes with it. It is helpful to guide children to become interested in the details of the way the air comes in and goes out, and in the involuntary physical movements that accompany it.

No forcing should ever be used with the breath, and deeper physical relaxation can be encouraged with each exhalation.

If children become agitated during the quiet focus it may be an indication that the time is not right for quiet work and they need some physical or emotional release. Sometimes they may need only a few encouraging and positive reminders to keep trying with the inner focus.

Breath awareness exercise
Humming through the middle of me

Age range: 8 years to adult.
1 Ask children to sit comfortably on chairs or cushions.
2 *Visualise a tunnel going inside you from the top of your head, down to the chair or cushion.*
3 *Breathe a full breath in without forcing at all.*
4 *On the out-breath let your body go soft and picture the air going down the tunnel, watching and feeling it all the way down.*
5 *Let's do this now for ten slow, full breaths.*
6 *Now hum as the breath goes down through you. Feel the humming going down that tunnel in the middle of you.*
7 Ask children to continue the exercise for about three or four minutes.
8 Ask children to express how they feel with a drawing and/or through a group discussion.

Quiet focusing: earthing

Earthing is the practice of focusing on sensation in the body, while dropping thoughts and allowing relaxation. This work needs lots of direction as children can easily find their thoughts wandering off. You can gently call them back to body awareness with simple directions such as presenting a progressive order of body parts for focusing awareness on (see page 90 for more details). These include breath, posture, and shifting awareness down into the belly, the centre of the body, etc. Body outline drawings are useful to guide this work and to survey the results (see *Emotional Release For Children* pages 64 and 65).

Awareness with touch

Working in pairs, use simple touch, stroking or massage to the hands, feet, head or shoulders. The one receiving has the task of keeping their attention under the touch. Receiving the touch, when carefully given, is usually very relaxing.

This simple touch can help the child to have a more conscious sense of his or her own body. Since the touch is carefully given it could be a very important aspect of healing and developing trust. This work involves both giving and receiving. This helps form a bond that supports further work.

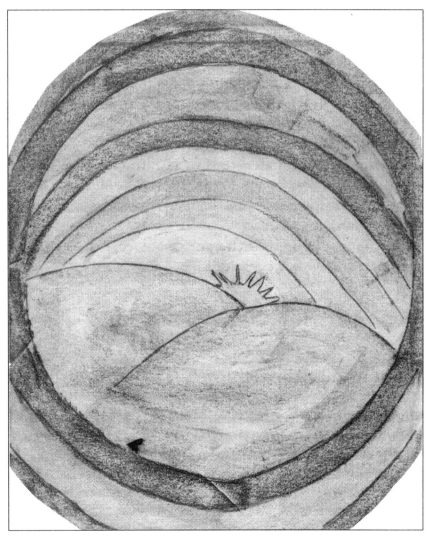

'I feel good now'
Mandala by an 8-year-old girl, after the exercise 'Humming through the middle of me'

Touch awareness exercise
The sounds inside

Age range: 6 years to adult.

Have drawing books and materials ready. The aim of this exercise is to support children with scattered, alive energy to focus and become centred.

1 Ask children to sit or kneel, with their body in an open position.
2 *Put your left hand gently on your throat and your right hand on your belly.*
3 *Take a moment to feel this from the inside.*
4 *Take a big breath in and then, on the out-breath let a big long sound come from your throat.*
5 *Move your left hand to your chest. Feel your hand resting there.*
6 *Take another big breath and let a sound come from your chest.*
7 *Try this a few times.*
8 Ask children to explore sounds that come from throat, chest, diaphragm, belly and forehead while repeating the full breaths.
9 On the second round ask them to make three fast sounds.
10 Then ask them to become still and quiet with their left hand on their chest and their right hand still on their belly, feeling the contact from inside themselves and being still.
11 Ask children to keep their eyes closed and 'see' what colours, lines, etc. would show the feeling inside their chest and belly.
12 Children finish the exercise by drawing the feeling inside their chest and belly.
13 Talk as a group about the differences before and after the exercise.

Coming home with rocking

This partner work is an excellent, gentle way to help children drop any muscular holding and stiffness from the day. Children lie on the floor and close eyes if that is comfortable. They take a few deep breaths, hold them for a moment, then relax. The partner gently places hands on the belly, saying what they are going to do, to avoid a shock. The partner then gently moves their hands back and forth. After a while, the hands can move up and down the body, rocking it from side to side. Children should be asked how they feel to make sure they are not frightened or nauseous. They should be invited to breathe fully and let the body go floppy.

Visualisations (see also page 100)

The following exercise is an example of a visualisation that supports self-awareness and relaxation.

Visualisation exercise for relaxation
An iceberg in the tropics

Age range: 8 years to adult.
Have drawing books and materials ready.
This exercise is useful for relaxing all the muscles of the body. It is important to give instructions slowly.

1 *Lie down, relax, close your eyes. Take three big slow breaths.*

2 *Picture yourself as an iceberg floating in the Arctic Ocean. It is very cold there. An iceberg is a huge chunk of ice, sometimes as big as a city building, floating in the ocean. It is usually very big, with just its tip rising above the water. You are the iceberg now.*

3 *You are floating towards the warm tropics. In the tropics it is very warm. There are palm trees and beautiful beaches. The sun becomes very hot. It beats down now on that part of you that is above the water. And the ocean is warming up too!*

4 *You know what happens when ice is in the sun. What happens as you—the iceberg—melt away? What does it feel like to join up with the ocean? Imagine yourself melting now. Imagine that the water in you, that was frozen, is now warm and blends in with the whole ocean. (Pause)*

5 *Have you melted away completely? Anything left?*

6 *Check if your arms are melted. Your legs? Belly?*

7 *Stay like that for a while. (Pause)*

8 *Now slowly move a little and slowly let your eyes open and come back into this room.*

9 Invite children to draw what it felt like to be melted.

10 Make discussion time available, possibly using the drawings as a starting point.

11 Creative writing could follow the experience of the exercise, drawing, and discussion.

Floppy limbs

Each child lies on the floor with limbs spread out. One by one the partner lifts each limb, gives it a gentle shake. Invite children to let their bodies go floppy.

Each limb is put down with gentle vibration and a very slight traction (stretching). The head is gently lifted and turned a little from side to side, with the instruction *Let your head rest in my hand, don't hold it up, don't help me, let your head go heavy*. This can be repeated several times. Feedback is invited so that partners can adjust how they work.

Autogenic phrases

These suggest certain states to the body. Suggesting relaxation can bring it about as the muscular system responds to the images. These phrases can be a good introduction to relaxation. They can be used by parents for children who are tired and would go to sleep wound up. The phrases can be made up to invite the body to soften, melt, open, relax, become warm—especially the belly, chest and face.

The word 'relaxation' has little meaning for younger children but the images of *melting like an ice cream* or of becoming *soft like a bunny* do.

Awakening the senses

Exercises that open imagination through the five senses can be incorporated into several subject areas, especially the sciences. Here are some suggestions to help you create your own exercises.

1 Before doing focused awareness with the senses, begin with dearmouring the body, focused body movements (for example, structured dance), and very few words.

2 Follow with a quiet time to stretch the ability to watch and wait. Invite children to listen to their insides: breath, heartbeat, tingling of energy.

3 Create experiences of:
   • looking and seeing clearly
   • using touch alone
   • exploring textures
   • hearing without naming the sounds or seeing the source of the sound
   • smelling
   • tasting—sweet, sour, salty, etc.

For example:
• Children could sit in a beautiful garden or natural bushland. Alternate earthing (see page 90) with eyes closed and then with eyes opened to allow the visual impressions to flood in.

• Children could sit in the playground at school with blindfolds on, simply listening without naming the in-coming sounds.

• Children are blindfolded. Give them fresh herbs to crush and smell. They could be asked what images or colours come to their mind with the different scents, or to find adjectives that go with the scent.

Relaxation exercise with autogenic phrases

Inviting softness

Age range: 8 years to adult.
Soft, carpeted space for lying down is essential.
It is important to give instructions slowly.

1 *Picture a warm sunny day. You are lying in the shade on soft warm grass. Your whole body feels happy and relaxed. Your body is warm and comfortable. It feels just right. Wriggle your body a little and feel the grass underneath. It is a quiet day and there is nothing you have to do now. You have time to be comfortable, relaxed and warm. Feel your head resting on the grass. Feel your back. Your back is getting soft, relaxed, warm. Your arms can spread out a bit. Now your body feels open like a flower, wide like the beach. Your legs are warm and comfortable. They are relaxing. Your legs can be strong and soft at the same time. They sometimes feel like tiger's legs. Now they can be still and melt a bit into the grass. Begin to feel your strength and feel how good it is to relax. Your body is warm and comfortable, soft and open.*

2 Guide children to bring their awareness back into the room gradually.

3 Invite children to look around the room, or out the window, or through scrap magazines, to find images that correspond to their relaxed state, for example, a willow tree, a bird soaring through the sky, the clouds.

4 Ask children to draw or create a collage about softness.

5 Follow with a group discussion on softness—and possibly its relationship to strength—based on children's experience and their drawing or collage.

Sensory awareness exercise
Using my nose instead of my eyes

Age range: 8 years to adult.

Prepare three bowls of strong-smelling herbs for each small group, for example, cloves, bay leaves, garam masala, basil, cinnamon bark.

Have drawing books and crayons ready with three circles drawn on one page.

Have quiet, relaxing music in the background.

If working in groups ask children to sit in circles of 3 or 4.

1 Ask children to close their eyes and place a bowl of herbs in the middle of each group.

2 *Let your eyes close. Tune in to your body. Take some deep breaths. Let your hand reach out and feel for bowl. Take a few of the herbs from it.*

3 *Crush the herbs between your fingers. Breathe in the aroma. Let your whole self sink into the world of the smell.*

4 *See how it makes you feel. Does it bring an 'Oh Yes' or a 'No'? Is it a comfortable or uncomfortable smell?*

5 *Take another breath in. Let the aroma come into you. Keep your eyes closed so that you can concentrate on the smell. Be still and quiet now.*

6 *Is it exciting? Is it boring?*

7 *What happens in your mind? Does the smell remind you of anything? Are you trying to guess what the herb is?*

8 *What happens in your body as the smell comes in? Does it bring an opening or a closing. Do you like it?*

9 *Can you stay with the smell and let it be your whole world for a moment? Simply be very still and quiet and use your nose.*

10 *Are there any feelings the smell reminds you of? See if any pictures or places come to mind, perhaps a scene you know or one that your imagination is making. Let the smell inspire your imagination. What sort of a landscape would go with that smell? Inland? Coastal? Desert? Rainforest? Another planet? Perhaps some place from the past or the future? A high place? A low place? Is it a place you know or a place you would like to go to?*

11 *What colours would go with this smell?*

12 *Do any particular words come with this smell or experience? Are there three words that sum up how you respond to the smell?*

13 *Draw the pictures or colours that came into your mind in the first circle. Around the edge of the circle write any words that came to mind.*

14 Repeat the process with the other two herbs.

15 Share drawings, words and inner experiences.

Vision quest

A vision quest is a time spent with nature that offers participants many challenges. There may be the rugged demands of walking, fasting and camping out away from the comforts of everyday life. This experience can bring an improved connection with a more essential self and stimulation of creativity. Vision quest exercises are most suitable for adolescents. Finding stillness in natural surroundings also supports the finding of inner stillness. Presenters need to be well prepared and to have addressed all safety issues.

A vision quest is ideal for adolescents as it offers challenges that can activate their inner resources: intelligence, cooperation, awareness, etc. In planning a vision quest the aim is to create an adventure that puts participants back in touch with inner direction, guidance and the will to carry out their intent.

Remember outer stillness usually highlights the incessant inner movement of chattering minds. Do not demand any long periods of sitting still. Modern children may need exercises such as long bushwalks to use up any overactive physical energy; this is very healthy and stops their mind grabbing onto the energy and turning it into nervous excitement.

Vision quest exercise
The ascent of the mountain

Age range: 12 years to adult.
This is an advanced group exercise for those who have already explored centring. It must be conducted outdoors in a beautiful place, with a real mountain or hill and, ideally, a wide view. Note that:

- Written parental consent will be necessary.
- Presenters must explore the area beforehand.
- Participants will need walking shoes, a thick towel to use as a cushion, warm clothes, journal, biro, snacks for after the quest.

An overview of the exercise, with clear safety rules, should be given before setting out.

The ascent
The quest begins at the foot of the mountain.

1 Begin in silence. Gather together, then proceed in convoy with one person clearly designated to lead and someone else chosen to stay at the end of the group.

2 Walk slowly, with frequent brief periods of stillness to look around and fully appreciate the natural setting.

Note: Awareness can be brought to the feet as in Zen walking (see page 78).

The summit

3 At the top, or designated meditation area, everyone finds 'their spot' to sit, within sight of the presenter, and preferably facing a wide view. Towels are used as cushions.

4 Everyone should close their eyes and their bodies relax in a sitting position. This is the time to find an inner centre.

5 Children should alternate opening eyes and taking in the view without speaking, and closing eyes and centring.

6 Guide children to work towards centring within and allowing the view to come in so that their attention is divided between the outside and inside.

7 After about fifteen minutes invite children to ponder one important question such as:
  - *What is really important to me?*
  - *Is there something my inner self is trying to tell me?*
  - *How should I deal with a specific problem in my life now?*

8 After about 15 minutes pondering, children journal their thoughts, decisions and new questions.

9 They thank 'their spot' and nature for supporting them.

The descent

10 Give a visual signal to the children to gather in silence.

11 Walk slowly down the track in convoy, focusing inner awareness in the heart.

Integration

12 After the descent and the formal end to the quest, gather for discussion, sharing and snacks.

Magic power animal

This is a way to allow identification of energies and impulses within so that children can be opened up to self-esteem and personal empowerment. The animals are used to project inner aspects that may not be consciously known.

Power animal visualisation exercise
Finding my power animal

Age range: 8 years to adult.

Have drawing books and materials ready.

Enthusiasm for the exercise can be greatly increased if some sort of 'canoe' can be put together, for example with bean bags, cushions, chairs, or simply a space marked out on a carpeted floor. Children sit or kneel in this space.

Note: If the exercise is being conducted in the classroom, some of the movement and sounding steps can be left out. However, there will be more benefit if the body is involved.

1 *We are going to take an imaginary canoe ride to a mysterious island.*

2 *First we must build the canoe. Gather those cushions/chairs and, all together, figure out how to make a canoe.* (Pause while they build)

3 *Good, now all get in, push it off. Feel it rise up over that wave.*

4 *Let's all row together, across the ocean.* (Invite actions or visualisation.)

5 *Now we are at the island. Wait quietly for a moment, you will see an animal appear.*

6 *There are many friendly animals on this island. One of them has been waiting just for you. It will come to you soon. Be very still and relaxed now.*

7 *See it coming. Look at every detail of it.*

8 *Make friends with your animal, pat it.* (Pause)

9 *Let it be close to you. It is a special, safe animal.*

10 Now it is giving you its power. Feel its animal strength coming inside you. (Pause)

11 Now it says goodbye. It tells you that it will always be with you, inside you.

12 Let this animal energy, that is now inside you, move and dance a bit. Let yourself move like the animal now.

13 Think about its sound. Now make its sound. Let it make its sound with your voice.

14 Now come back to the canoe. It is time to row home.

15 Push the canoe off the beach. Feel it rise again over the waves.

16 Now we row home.

17 Invite children to draw themselves as the animal, or make a mask of it, to remind them of its strength and help.

18 You could follow with a discussion on ways that the animal's power would be helpful in children's lives.

19 Children could find a feather, claw, hairs or other object as a way of remembering the animal.

Self-awareness

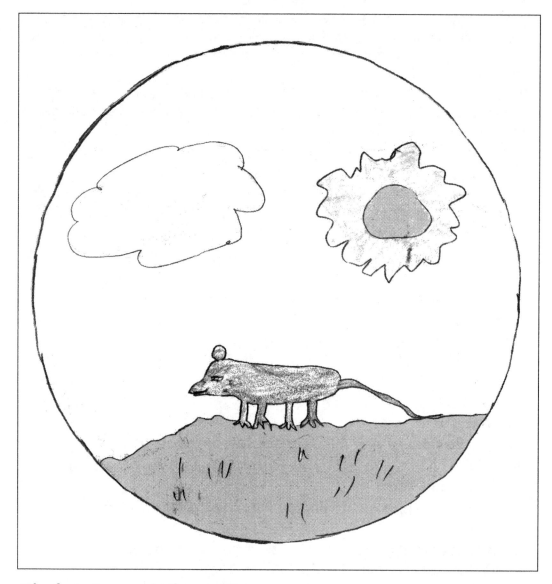

'The fastest mouse in the world'
Drawn by a 9-year-old boy after the exercise 'Finding my power animal'

Self-awareness exercise
Looking inside myself

Age range: 8 years to adult.
The aim of this exercise is to:

- gather inner knowledge that will improve communication skills
- locate problem areas/symptoms in the body
- bring deeper self-awareness
- bring relaxation and ability to turn within.

Have body outline drawings and crayons ready.

1 Invite children to lie down on cushions or carpet and close their eyes.

2 Ask them to take a few deep breaths and relax.

3 Guide children to imagine they are very little and can go inside themselves to check through each part of the body.

4 *You are very very little and have a torch. You are so small that we can hardly see you. Imagine you are inside yourself now, that you can just slide inside. You are going to check around inside to see what is there, to see what you can discover. You are beginning inside your head, shining the torch around inside. You move gradually from your head down through your body to your toes. Imagine you are walking through a tunnel inside you.*

5 *Now return your awareness to your forehead. As you walk around in there you find a control room, like the control tower at an airport, where you can see all the rest of your insides. There is a radar in this room and it is switched on. It can sweep through the body to find things. The radar will sweep through and look for these things. If it finds them, you turn over and draw them on the body outline beside you. Pretend that is a map of you. You will need to feel what colours and what lines feel just right to describe what the radar finds.*

6 Things the radar looks for (take time to look for each one):
- coldness, coolness
- heat or warmth
- weakness
- strength
- relaxed, free, light parts
- tight, holding, tense parts
- busy or troubled parts
- peaceful parts.

7 Ask children to show the completed body outline drawing to you or a partner and describe what was found. They might consider showing it to parent/s.

8 Try to draw out conversation that may enlarge on children's self-awareness and some possible causes for what was found.

Note: After children have worked with meditation for some time you can see changes when reviewing the body outline drawings. For older children, review of their body outline drawings will confirm their own growth.

Self-awareness exercise

Using colour and movement to find a gift inside

Age range: 10 years to adult.

This exercise has three parts. You decide whether to use the second two parts. Watch the attention span of the children and the depth to which they can go into themselves. Most adolescents will resist the movement part. When you explore this exercise for yourself ask a friend to read out the instructions.

You need a large space for free movement.

Have a large blank page and crayons ready in front of each child.

Part one: Using colour

1 Ask children to sit quietly on their own with paper and crayons. Give instructions slowly so that you keep pace with the children.

2 *When you begin to draw start at the top of the page.*

3 *Close your eyes. Feel inside, listen to what is inside you: the feelings and energy.*

4 *Take several big breaths.*

5 *Open your eyes now. Choose the right colour for how it feels inside you.*

6 *Draw a line that goes with how you feel. Look at it. Is it exactly right?*

7 *If it is not right do another line or choose another colour and try again. See if you can get closer to showing how you really feel. Since you have begun to tune in, there will be change.*

8 *Keep going, drawing lines until you get to the bottom of the page.*

9 *There may be a word that goes with your feeling. Feel the energy with which you draw. Let your feelings continue to be in the energy, in your hand. Let the drawing help you know exactly how you feel.*

10 *Ask yourself: where is all this happening in me? If it looks wrong, turn the page and keep going.*

11 *Keep tuning in. Are the lines heavy enough? Light enough?*

12 *Are there one or two words for your inner picture? Write them.*

Part two: Adding movement

13 Ask children to take the drawing to an open, clear space and stand in front of it.

14 *Find the posture or stance that goes with the drawing.*

15 *Close your eyes. See if any part of your body wants to move in response to your drawing.*

16 *Let some movement start. Let it change and grow.*

17 *Find a sound that goes with the colours. Try out a few sounds. Which one feels right to you? Make the sound a few times.*

18 *Let the movement increase. Let it be tighter, faster, slower, more flowing, more of what it is! Is it more of a regular beat or wilder?*

19 *Let your energy express itself fully. Let the sound grow. Put your whole body into it!* (Pause)

20 *Now let yourself melt down onto the floor, go floppy and still.*

21 *There is nothing to do now. Can you open your mind to receive some images from inside?*

Part three: A gift from inside

22 *Stay very still. Can you feel things moving inside?*

23 *Watch inside yourself and let an image, a picture or memory come. Don't try too hard; let the picture come to you.*

24 *When you see it, look carefully. There might be one thing, many things.*

25 *When you are in touch with what you have received, gently sit up. Don't talk or look around too much yet.*

26 *Draw what you saw in your special book or journal.*

27 *Pick someone to be your partner and tell them about your experience.*

28 After discussion, support children to explore their own meanings for the images through some simple Gestalt steps:
   • *Close your eyes again,*
   • *feel inside yourself, and then say:*
     'I am ...' (description of your image)
     My purpose is ...' (See page 150 for more details.)

29 Encourage children to write down what they have learned.

Visualisation exercise

Your dream home
(from Dorothy Bottrell)

Age range: 12 to 18 years.
Have writing materials ready.

1 Begin with relaxation melt-down, by taking breath and attention to each part of the body, then to the whole body.

2 *Allow a picture to come into your mind. You are standing outside a house. It is your new house, the one you designed and built exactly how you wanted it. Notice the location. Where is your house? Is it in the city or the country? Near the beach? Is it a noisy, busy place, or quiet and secluded?*

3 *Your new home is almost ready for you to move in. Some things are unfinished, but most of it is now complete. So go inside now and take a look around your home, your dream home.*

4 *Walk around each room and notice its colours, its features. Notice the details—the textures under your feet, the quality of light, the size and shape of the space of each room. Notice your own creative touch in each room, providing beauty along with all the essential features you needed. (Pause) Notice too, what still needs to be done to bring your home to completion.*

5 *As you come back to awareness of being in this room and feeling the floor/chair beneath you, allow the images of each room to stay with you. Tune in again to your body and notice the feelings inside, in your muscles, your bones, in each area of your body, in your heart. Be aware again of how you are breathing and direct your breath down into your back.*

6 *Now take your attention to your legs. Take a deep breath that brings your energy right down into your legs, your feet, your toes. Which room of your house belongs with your legs? Just let the image come into your mind.*

7 *Now take your attention to your stomach, taking three deep breaths, right down into your belly. What room belongs there?*

8 *Now, to the head. Take your awareness to your head, your neck, your face. Which room goes with the feelings in your head? Use your mind's eye to notice the details again.*

9 *Finally, take three deep breaths into your chest, the heart area. Feel the expansion, the openness of that part of your body. The heart, the focus of giving and receiving love. Notice how it feels now. Which room goes with that feeling? Which room is the heart of your home?*

10 *Stay in this relaxed position. In a few moments I'll ask you to open your eyes and write down a few things so you can remember the images that came to you. Stay quiet, stay with how you feel now.*

Write down which room went with which part of your body and then describe any details you remember about each room.

11 Open your eyes now and write about the room you associated with your back, your legs, your belly, your head, and your heart.

12 Describe the rooms.

13 For each room complete this statement: 'I am like this room because ...'

14 Write about what was unfinished in your home? Are you like this in any way?

15 Write about how you feel now.

Relaxation

Relaxation is about letting go, about managing ourselves in a better way. If you find children are too agitated to work with the exercises, you could suggest that the school counsellor try some of the release exercises in *Emotional First-Aid For Children* and *Emotional Release For Children*. These address the emotional causes of much stress and tension and deal with a deeper level of emotional healing work.

The ideas and exercises included here address the need to:

• take time to recognise the depths of stresses and tensions

• find methods to allow tension to drop away

• find how to live without this chronic tension.

Have you ever met anyone over the age of about 15 who considered himself or herself to be relaxed enough? Adults tend to have more stress than children. This increase in stress accompanies more responsibility and self-awareness. It seems in our culture that the age when stress symptoms begin to show up is becoming younger and younger. Stress reduction and stress management classes in secondary schools are proving a boon to those children facing exams or finding life just too much.

Most of us can identify activities that we find relaxing. Do we enjoy them often enough? To create an atmosphere that is conducive to relaxation consider what helps you relax. Does your list of activities and environments include any of these: warm baths, sitting by the ocean, having quiet about you, listening to music, lying down, watching clouds, trees and birds and nature, hugging, rocking, massaging, sitting by a fire, playing with pets, floating in water, dancing, playing a musical instrument? How could some of these be translated into activities, visualisations or aspects of the environment?

Preparing to teach relaxation

Choosing methods for relaxation will depend on a number of factors.

Attention span of the children: It is vital to invite stillness and never to force anything if a child is to continue into relaxation. If stillness is impossible then restless energy may have to be expressed strongly in order to leave a clearer space inside, for example through bioenergetics, brisk walking.

There is an obvious connection between age and attention span. Younger children will usually exhibit a shorter attention span. Extending the attention span will be influenced by any previous experience with inner-life skills. A willingness to be quiet and attentive usually increases with an experience of the benefits of the exercises.

Amount of time available: This will determine the depth of the relaxation possible, as well as the number of stages of the exercise that can be included.

Time of day: Mornings are times for aliveness whereas afternoons tend to be natural times of low energy. Dusk is a natural time for quietness, as nature around us begins to settle for the night. You also need to be aware of personal rhythms, and discuss these with children. For example: *Are you a 'morning person'? A 'night owl'?*

Current need: Is the relaxation work a spontaneous need? a parental need? the child's need? A crisis? Part of a regular program?

State of the presenter: The work will go well if the method used corresponds to the presenter's experience and understanding. What has helped you most to relax? Which exercises are you most comfortable with?

State of the children: Children can come to the exercises in various states of excitement, lethargy, willingness or resistance. This may determine the type of work suitable for them, for example, strong or gentle, fast or slow, etc.

Location: Is there lots of space? Are there outer distractions? Can full expression be allowed, that is, lots of noise? Will there be amusing or distracting noises or voices from the environment when the children are quiet? Can the room be darkened or lights dimmed to aid relaxation?

Space available: Will children be sitting? Standing? Is there room to lie down? Is it comfortable to lie down?

Is it group or individual work? In group work it is more difficult to find the right length of time, as there will be a range of attention spans. With individuals it is clear how long the person can sustain relaxation and be still before they start twitching, wriggling, scratching or opening eyes and looking around.

Children's readiness to go through the transition: Allow them to peek about, giggle and express any discomfort they may have before moving from familiar games, activities or lessons to inner-life skills work.

Stages in relaxation work

When doing relaxation work you will find it useful to work through the following steps:

1 Set the work space and make it private. Create order. You could have an arrangement of beautiful objects, and perhaps candles, in the centre of the work space or on a table or shelf. Dimmed lights help eyes relax.

2 Give an overview of the exercise and the reasons for doing it.

3 Release any initial agitation with, for example, brisk walking, shaking, bioenergetics, sounding and some deep breaths.

4 Deal with the issue of trust, and any resistance or embarrassment at doing inner focus work.

5 Guide attention to turn within to the sensations of the body—'what is there inside'.

6 Follow structure for the relaxation sequence. For example, will the relaxation sequence move around the limbs? Down through the centre of the body?

7 Be ready to give direction to guide the children's attention and call it back when distracted.

8 Use imagery and story. Imagery can help convey the sense of relaxation, for example: *floppy like a puppy asleep, soft like melted cheese on a pizza.* See stories pages 59–60.

9 Introduce stillness and silence, that is, some time in the exercise where nothing is said or done. The length of this time will depend on the experience of the group with the inner-life skills.

10 Invite private expression of experiences through drawing, writing, modelling, choosing symbols to represent the experience, etc.

11 Ask children to share experiences through listening to others and asking questions.

Relaxation exercise
What is here now?

Age range: 12 years to adult.

Part one

1 If possible ask children to lie down on a carpeted floor with a cushion under their head and close their eyes. However, sitting in a relaxed, balanced posture in chairs will also work.

2 *Remember yourself at home early this morning, and visualise all the things you were doing. Visualise each step up until now.*

3 *Follow each step, each feeling of your day until now, as if mentally watching a home video. (Give more guidance to younger children.)*

4 *Feel your body and its energy now.*

Part two

5 *Focus on your energy. What does it feel like? Is it mostly in your head? In your thoughts? In a part of your body?*

6 *Is there a feeling of being 'at home' in your chest? Belly? Hands? Legs?*

7 *Spend a few minutes to drop all your thinking. Is this possible?*

8 *Allow your body to relax more, to go floppy, to melt.*

9 *Watch. Become a watcher who looks inside, who simply observes what is inside your body.*

10 *Let your awareness come to your breath, let it relax.*

11 *Let your awareness keep dropping down with each breath into your body. Let it drop into the middle of yourself, like your mind was sliding into a tunnel that is through the middle of you.*

12 *Every time you think about something else, come back down inside this tunnel in you.*

Part three

13 After about 5 or 10 minutes bring the children's attention back to the surroundings; invite their breath to deepen.

14 Invite children to quietly sit up and stretch.

15 Ask them to draw the tunnel, the colours, the shapes, what it was like inside.

16 Invite them to share the experience.

Note: For younger children add more imagery; make your guidance more of a story.

Relaxation exercise using visualisation
A fern in the forest

Age range: 7 to 12 years.
Have drawing books and materials ready.
Have soft, relaxing music in the background (see page 154).

1 Ask children to stand and:
 • close their eyes (if they are comfortable with that)
 • become still
 • take a few big breaths and sigh out. Invite them to imagine the scene following and act out the story.

2 *Imagine you are a young fern, still unfolding, still growing, still uncurling. It is a bright new morning. There are patches of sunshine, patches of shade.*

3 *See the clearing around you. See the grass, the trees, the colours, the shapes. Hear the birds and the breeze gently blowing through the trees.*

4 *This breeze is beginning to make you sway and dance gently. This breeze keeps changing directions. You are bending. You are flexible. You are alive with gentle movements, your roots are in the earth but you are dancing free in the breeze.*

5 *Take some full breaths and sigh out.*

6 *In this warmth your fronds, your tender new branches are beginning to unfold. They are spreading out to receive the warmth.*

7 *Some ants are suddenly running up your side! Feel them tickle. Shake them off if you want to.*

8 *The breeze has stopped. Now be still. Picture the grass and trees, birds and warmth and breathe this into you. Feel your full size.*

9 *See in your mind's eye what you are part of, what you the fern are connected to, what is around you.*

10 *Feel the sap rising up from the ground, up through the centre of you to the tiny leaves at your tips.*

11 *Imagine what you would look like to a bush walker. (Pause) Now gently come back to being yourself.*

12 Direct children to draw themselves as the fern in the forest.

13 Ask children to talk about their experience of the exercise.

Gestalt role-play exercise could be used as a follow-up (see page 150).

Relaxation exercise
Visualising relaxation

Age range: 12 years to adult.

This sequence is based on the Alexander Technique which uses both physical relaxation and visualisation to assist the body to let go, assume its natural posture and come to a quiet state.

1 Ask children to lie on their backs, on a carpeted floor with a cushion or books under their head. This keeps the neck lengthened and the head supported. Knees should be kept up with feet flat on the carpet, in a balanced position. Children's arms are by their sides, with hands resting on their sides.

2 *Imagine your neck is going floppy and growing longer.*

3 *Let your trunk be free to lengthen and widen. Picture this happening. Imagine or think this rather than doing it.*

4 *Feel your chest and belly. Give them permission to let go now, to melt down like an ice block on a hot day.*

5 *Visualise your shoulders going apart from each other. Allow your body to follow this image.*

6 *Tune into your belly. Is anything tight? Let go in your belly now.*

7 *Imagine your legs letting go from the hips, as if the joints were softer. Then imagine this happening in your hips.*

8 *It is quite likely that you will find your body taking some full breaths so encourage this.*

9 *Imagine your legs moving up towards the ceiling, in the direction your knees are pointing. A tiny magic force is at work! Feel what it is doing inside you.*

10 *Check through from head to toes. Could any parts do with some more melting?*

11 *Stay like this for a little while. Feel what it is like inside you now.* (Pause)

12 *Slowly wiggle your toes a little and stretch your fingers.*

13 *Turn onto your side, curl up for a moment.*

14 *Now gently sit up.*

15 *Gather with two others and talk about how you feel now and what you thought of the exercise.*

16 Follow the exercise with group discussion on the different experiences of the body before and after the exercise.

Visualisation stories for relaxation
Creating trust and serenity

Age range: 8 years to adult.

These visualisation stories work best after some energetic release work. Children are invited to watch the images and action of the story in their mind's eye.

Ask children to lie down or rest in a comfortable position, ideally with their eyes closed.

Note: Use only one story at a time. After each story use the usual integration steps of drawing, discussion and writing.

1 The garden

You are in a beautiful garden on a fine warm day. Your friends and family are playing nearby, but you are by yourself in this part of the garden. There are tall trees, green bushes around you and lots of bright flowers. Birds are flying about and singing in the trees.

- *You are lying on your back on the warm soft grass.*

- *You have been watching the trees moving in the breeze. You see the branches bend and dance as the leaves flutter above everything. Sometimes you even wish you could be riding up there on those branches.*

- *Behind the trees you see blue sky and white clouds. Now you watch the clouds drift by. As they float across the sky they change shape. Watch your clouds now. What shapes are they making? Do the shapes remind you of anything?*

- *Now listen to the birds. They sing to each other. There is one above you now, can you see it? It is singing just for you. What do you think it would say if it could sing in human language?*

- *The bird has been called away by other birds. You are resting warm and comfortable on the grass. You close your eyes. You can feel the warm air on your skin and deep inside you feel your heart beating. You rest like this for a moment.*

2 The full moon

It is a warm evening. You are on a camping trip with your best friends. It is past your bedtime but you are not tired. There is a full round moon, reflecting a silver-white light over the bush around you. Your friends are nearby, but they are not talking. You have just cooked a meal together on the camp fire, eaten it, chatted for a while, and now you are lying in your sleeping bag, watching the night.

- *The flames of the fire leap up. They look bright in the darkness. Watch in your mind's eye the colours of yellow and orange and red flames. Keep watching the flames for a while. (Pause)*

- Now look up to the sky. There are no clouds and you can see millions of planets and stars. As you watch the stars you imagine joining them up, drawing lines from one to another, until they make huge pictures above you.

- As you listen you can hear insects singing. They seem to be glad of the darkness as they call to each other.

- Your sleeping bag is soft. The air is warm. You relax and rest.

3 The mountain stream

It is a fresh spring morning. You are on a bushwalk with friends. You are walking a little behind them, enjoying nature. You are wearing your old sneakers as you walk up along a stream, splashing through the shallow parts. You move in and out of the sun under the shadows of the trees that line the stream.

- You look about at the trees. Some have been knocked over by floods. Some are new and young and straight. There are many shades of green in the leaves and the grass around you.

- As you stroll along you can hear the sound of the water flowing over the stones. Listen to the sound of the water. Is it saying anything to you? (Pause)

- You can hear birds singing in the trees above. Listen to them now. (Pause)

- You sit for a while on a smooth warm rock at the water's edge. Your feet are in the cool flowing stream. Now you lie back on the warm rock.

- Beside you are two lizards sunning themselves. They are the same colour as the rock. They are staying very still.

- Take a few deep breaths of the country air and relax. Rest here for a while.

CHAPTER FIVE

Practising freedom, grace and beauty

Freedom, grace and beauty are the natural
attributes of every animal organism.
Freedom is the absence of inner restraint to
the flow of feeling, grace is the expression
of this flow in movement, while beauty is a
manifestation of the inner harmony such a
flow engenders. They denote a healthy
body and also, therefore, a healthy mind.

Alexander Lowen, *Bioenergetics*

Emotional and physical release as preparation

Sometimes you simply have to break free of tension and frustration before enjoying quiet times or inner focus. Children often need to free the tension of held emotions or incomplete grief or anger, for example, before agreeing to meditation. Exercises that bring release through shaking, shouting, dancing and running can help with this, although it may not necessarily be welcome in every setting. Many teachers book the school hall for this work, or march the children briskly down to the oval or play area, away from other classes.

Since many children carry a burden of emotional stress, there may be a need for some emotional release. They may need to face the wall and 'tell off' people they are angry with. They might need to 'get it off their chest' before being ready for more subtle self-awareness. Bioenergetics and dearmouring games are helpful here. The ones used in ERC have been freely adapted from the work of Drs Alexander Lowen and John Pierrakos in the USA (see *Emotional Release For Children* pages 97–99, 113, 116).

Sometimes a child's energy for living enthusiastically has been depressed. This can result in disinterest in daily activities, emotional depression, muscular aches and pains. Games that draw attention to this held body energy and then assist its release allow the feelings and energy to move again, to be expressed. This movement can bring healing and a sense of harmony, peace and renewed creativity.

Some exercises intentionally bring stress to the body for a moment in order to make muscles let go (as you do in massage). For example: *See how long you can hold your arms up in the air.* Once the body relaxes and the energy moves again, emotions can flow and release will happen if it is needed. Then there is a clear state for inner focus.

Our way of using bioenergetic exercises, sometimes supported by rhythmic music and the principles of meditation, creates an activation in the body systems and energy. Individual sequences of exercises are designed to activate specific segments of the body. They begin a flow, a release and direct exploration of a specific feeling or make inner space for surrender and relaxation. The bioenergetics sequences usually begin with tuning-in within, meeting what is there already. All this work is stronger and more effective if children are already connected a little to their own state, mood, body energy.

Sometimes bioenergetics simply helps children 'let off steam', much like playground games and sport. They can also activate emotions that are close to the surface, so should only be offered when there is time and support for children to complete and integrate and feel closure.

Vibration, shaking and deliberate shivering are also used. These help break down the muscular holding and energy stasis. There seems to be a direct correlation to creative imagination and free flowing of energy. Try to encourage a state of surrender in children; this allows the body the freedom to do what it needs to do. It also avoids over-exertion and strain.

Expanding the breath is used throughout the active exercises. The breath can be chaotic or ordered, through the mouth or nose, and can be focused into chest, belly or whole torso. Sounding is included: either gently humming to stimulate energy, or cathartic and loud to release emotional flow and clear old patterns of holding in the throat and jaw. Sounding also reverses old childhood patterns of restricted expression.

Movement and stretching loosens muscles and joints so that they operate more freely. Mechanical expansion, including stretching limbs, spine and especially the chest, counters the unconscious contraction that stressed children have learnt, and now carry. Body weight and purposeful tension are sometimes used to 'over-work' muscles a little so that their subtle chronic spasms release and energy can be felt to vibrate through the limbs.

Rhythm is used to encourage stronger movement and surrender of old patterns. If children follow the rhythm in movement work, the holding can surrender. This is effective for children up to about thirteen or fourteen years. After this they are usually too self-conscious to participate. Sometimes inviting them to bring their own music to move to will overcome this awkwardness.

After physical activation and emotional clearing there is a need to have some time of stillness, to allow children to become deeply quiet. Children are invited to know themselves at the core, to watch within, to focus at the centre of the body.

Movement is also used after some exercises to complete, to integrate. In times of inner and outer freedom when the body's energy is very alive, the natural impulse with young children is to dance. Dance is a simple, creative expression that can bring a segment of work to a beautiful conclusion. Some young children find that they are really themselves when they are dancing.

Adolescents are usually inhibited about dancing in front of adults or others that they do not know. And, of course, the music chosen by adults is sure to be out of date for them!

Some of these exercises move from strong release movement to role-playing which can introduce a healthy element of fun. They proceed to slow motion, and then to stillness and visualisation. The aim of this progression is to invite peacefulness after using up the children's overactive or agitated energy in the first stages.

Preparation for quiet meditation

Basic bioenergetic exercises

Age range: 8 years to adult.

Acknowledge and accept any resistance or embarrassment and invite children to talk about this the first time they do these exercises.

Note: Always begin with a warm-up (as suggested in Step 1), then select three or four exercises to precede quiet work or simple stillness. Children must not do any exercises or assume postures that are painful, or require endurance.

1 Warm-up: *Stretch, take full breaths, shake the body and make sounds, such as sighing, groaning, growling.*

2 Bound and free: *Cross arms around the body, cross legs and hold everything tight. Then release all at once and run on the spot, shaking any tightness out of the limbs and making sounds. Repeat this several times.*

3 Freeing the face: *Close eyes tightly, suck in breath, hold, then release and open face, open eyes. Open eyes wide, keep the head still and make large circular movements with the eyeballs.*

4 The arch: *Stand and place feet about 30 cm apart, bend the knees, rest hands lightly on the lower back. Gently lean back until eyes are facing towards the ceiling. Do not let the head fall back. Breathe deeply. Hold this for a few minutes.*

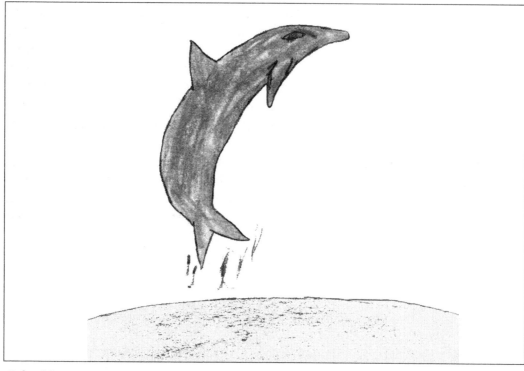

'I feel happy now'
Drawn by a 10-year-old boy, after the exercise 'Basic bioenergetic exercises'

5 The coiled spring: *Work in pairs. One child stands behind with hands on the shoulders of the other and begins to push down. The one experiencing the exercise allows knees to bend and allows himself to be pushed down until he doesn't like it, then springs up and stretches the limbs wide.*

6 Kicking: *Kick a cushion around the room. If working in pairs, one child holds a cushion up in the air and the other kicks, releasing sounds along with the kick.* (The one holding the cushion takes care to hold it at the side and avoid being in the way of the kicking!)

7 How strong is the wall? *Press with flat palms against a strong wall, gradually engaging the ankles, legs, lower back, shoulders, arms, hands, then the whole body. Keep the breathing full and free. Then relax for a moment.* (Repeat three times.)

8 The walk: *Walk in a large circle around the room, keeping hips free. This movement can be exaggerated for a while.*

9 Stillness: *Lie on the carpeted floor for a few minutes, keeping as still as possible. Direct the awareness within.*

Bioenergetic games to prepare for meditation

Age range: 8 to 12 years.

These stories or scenes for acting out are designed for younger children to support the release of frustrations or agitations. Encourage as much sound and action as you can. In some cases acting out several of the games might be helpful before attempting quieter work. Complete the games by moving directly into quiet meditations, or simply invite the children to draw how it felt to do the role play.

1 The twister

You are a mighty wind that blows around in circles. You blow around and around. You swirl around on yourself, collecting up things in the countryside around you. Show this with your arms. You make a loud swooshing noise. People are running away from you. You are very strong. You spin and spin. Then you stop. Let yourself collapse now. Be still for a moment.

2 The volcano

Picture yourself as an active volcano. From deep down inside there is pressure from the molten rock. This lava is pushing up against a plug at the top. Take a position that helps you feel a bit like the volcano. Act out the pressure inside the volcano, show this with your muscles. Now push up. Suddenly the plug in the top breaks loose and the lava shoots up with lots of colours and sounds. It flares up in all directions. Now you are the lava flowing down the side of the volcano. As the molten rock cools it flows more slowly. Soon it stops still.

3 The cheetah

You are a handsome cheetah, walking proudly through the jungle. You are quite hungry. Feel all those powerful muscles in your legs move as you walk along. Suddenly you see your friend ahead. You feel like playing. You begin to sneak up on him or her. You push through the long grass very slowly now. You plan to pounce and surprise your friend. Without being seen you move carefully and slowly into a good pouncing position. Now you tense every muscle in your body, getting ready to spring out of the long grass. You take in a deep breath. And now you pounce! You roll about with your friend and have a great game.

4 The snake

You are a beautiful big snake curled up on a warm rock. You have had a good lunch and you are enjoying the warmth. Your body is very relaxed as you curl around yourself. Suddenly the shadow of an eagle—your enemy—passes over you. You move away quickly to hide under the shelter of a rock. You are breathing fast after your fright. After a moment it is safe to come out. You slide back to the warm rock. Now you realise that your old skin feels too tight. You twist yourself about the rocks and begin to shed your old skin. Gradually each part of you wriggles across the rock to pull off the old dead skin. Now you are free of the tightness. Your body can relax and feel free. You decide to go for a swim to cool down. Your graceful movements make little waves through the water. Then you come back to dry and rest on the warm rock. Soon you fall asleep.

Active meditation

Tension and surrender

Age range: 7 years to adult.

This is a simple relaxation exercise to release deep tensions and is good to do before quiet work. It uses over-stressing to assist a deeper letting-go. Ideal for children who usually cannot keep still enough to do relaxation work.

1 Ask children to lie on a carpeted floor, stretch out limbs, contract and expand their bodies a few times.

2 Tell children to picture themselves as a five-pointed star, with each limb and the head as a point. They picture themselves floating, twinkling in a clear night sky.

3 Direct children to begin tensing body parts in this order:
   - *right hand, right arm, hold for a moment, let go*
   - *right foot, right leg, hold for a moment, let go*
   - *left foot, left leg, hold for a moment, let go*
   - *left hand, left arm, hold for a moment, let go*
   - *face, trunk, hold for a moment, let go.*

4 Establish a steady rhythm: (Tense! Tense! Hold! Relax!) Clap or use a drumbeat to help establish the rhythm.

5 Work through the list of body parts five or six times.

6 Give children time to lie still and invite them to feel themselves twinkling, pulsating as this star, with lots of quiet energy. Ask them to stay like this for a while being aware of any pictures that come into their mind's eye.

7 After the exercise children draw themselves as the star as a completing activity, or they can draw any image that came to them.

8 Children could now be guided into one of the quieter exercises.

Active meditation

Earth, water, fire, air and spirit

(From Paul Perfrement)

Age range: 14 years to adult.

This is an exercise for developing greater emotional balance and is based on various ancient traditions and the work of Jung.

This exercise uses five selections of music to support an inner experience and imagery related to the four elements. The inner experience is then related to self-awareness in daily life.

Have five selections of music ready. Choose these to support imagery of earth, water, air, fire and spirit.

Have a copy of the Four Element Sheet for each child, preferably enlarged to A3 size. (See page 156.)

Have crayons ready.

Part one: music experience

1 Ask children to stand, spread around the room. Ensure there is an arm's length distance between each child.

2 Place the Four Element Sheet and the crayons at their feet.

3 Make children aware of the four directions: south, west, north, east. Children can practise turning deliberately through the 90 degrees.

4 Children visualise themselves standing in the centre of their own circle. They stand for a moment, opening breath and feeling their feet on the floor.

5 Ask them to take one small step back to the southern edge of their circle.

6 Children close eyes and open to images from their imagination and memory of 'earth'.

7 Ask children to turn their attention deeply inside to see how they feel with the imagery and the music. Invite them to 'breathe in the music'.

8 Play earth music for about two minutes. If they wish to move with the music encourage this.

9 Ask children to quickly pick a coloured crayon that goes with the images and feeling when the music stops, and draw freely inside the 'earth circle' on the Four Element Sheet.

10 Ask children to stand and facing the same direction, slowly and deliberately turn 90 degrees to face the west.

11 Invite an image of water and play the second piece of music, etc. as above. The order of directions and elements is:
   - south—earth
   - west—water
   - north—air
   - east—fire.

12 Children then return to the centre of the circle after they have completed the exercise for all four directions/elements. They picture themselves at the centre—the point of interaction between all the elements and the centre of themselves.

13 Invite them to turn deeply within to focus on being open to the new within themselves—a place of acceptance, trust and openness to life or spirit while the music representing spirit is played.

14 Children then draw in the central circle on the sheet.

15 Encourage them to sit quietly in the centre of their circle for a few minutes with eyes closed.

16 Ask them to write one word, on the back of the sheet, that describes how they feel now.

Part two: integration, discussion and recording

17 Ask children to form small groups to share their experience.

18 Give them two or three open-ended questions to discuss. For example:
- *What happened? How did you feel before the exercise and now at the end?*
- *Was the experience different for each element?*
- *Did you feel stronger with any of the elements?*
- *Could what you learned apply to situations in your life?*

19 After some discussion ask the children to journal. Journal questions could include:
- *What parts of you are like air? Earth? Fire? Water?*
- *What element might you need more of in your life to achieve a greater balance?*
- *What element might you need to temper in your life?*
- *Describe what the experience of being open to life and spirit feels like to you, or means to you.*

20 *Perhaps one of the elements is very important for you now. How could you be more in touch with it in your daily life?*

Four Element Sheet
See Appendix 4 (page 156).

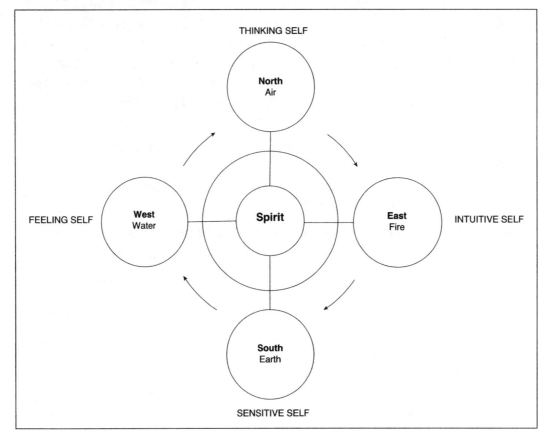

THINKING SELF

North
Air

FEELING SELF

West
Water

Spirit

East
Fire

INTUITIVE SELF

South
Earth

SENSITIVE SELF

Slow-motion movement

Moving in slow motion can be a great help in bringing awareness to the body and the energy within the body. Many of the exercises of Moshe Feldenkrais—*Awareness Through Movement* (1980)—utilise slow conscious movement as a way to build up a better connection with the body and to improve coordination. Slow motion is often used in the Eastern meditative exercises of Tai Chi and QiGong. The aim of these approaches to self-awareness is to become conscious of the body energy (Chi or Qi) through the movements and then to allow this energy to direct the movements. It is believed this brings emotional calm, clear thinking and good health.

If you seriously practise Tai Chi under the direction of an experienced teacher, you find that the slow movements and attempts to be graceful gradually allow the mind to slow down, the visual perception to sharpen and the body to relax. You feel more vital. The swirling repetitious thoughts begin to slow and you feel more whole. A positive emotional state emerges from this inner effort. All this makes learning easier.

The following exercises use slow motion to help the body relax and to prepare the way for effortless stillness. They can be worked with many times. Like all skills, the inner-life skills are learned through repeated efforts.

Active meditation
Moving in slow motion

Age range: 10 years to adult.

This exercise enhances body awareness. Keeping the movements at a very very slow speed forces the awareness to come into the limbs. This has a quietening effect on thoughts and feelings. Quiet flowing music will help (see Appendix 3).

Note: If children show signs of agitation during the slow-motion movement, pause and invite them to wriggle or shake, then start again. If their attention span is not sufficient to complete all steps of the exercise, just stop when it feels right, and go to step 12.

1 Ask children to lie on a carpeted floor on their backs, with limbs spread out.

2 *Close your eyes, take a few deep breaths and relax.*

3 *Leaving your arms resting on the carpet, begin turning your wrists very, very slowly—so slowly that the movement is between the point of stillness and movement.*

4 *There is nothing now but this movement. Feel the little changes in the muscles as the movement continues.*

5 *Leave the wrists now, and focus on and move your ankles. They can turn the same way, or opposite, it doesn't matter. Don't think about it, just feel the slow movement.*

6 *Work like this with your head, turning it slowly. Don't strain your neck.*

7 *Work with an ankle and a wrist from opposite sides of the body. Now change to the opposite wrist and ankle.*

8 *Add the head. Keep the head, ankle and wrist moving together very slowly. Don't think about it! Lose yourself in the slow motion.*

9 *Now slowly, gently kneel up. Let the upper part of your body turn through space—keep it slow!*

10 *Add the wrists and head, either all together or one at a time.*

11 *Slowly stand up and allow all parts to move together. Now add turning the whole body through space. Let go of all control now, surrender to the flowing. Just let everything move, flow, turn.*

12 *Now be still. Feel the stillness. Is it really stillness? Be inside yourself now. How would you describe it?* (Pause)

13 *Focus inside and think about what this energy would like to create. Imagine if there were no limits, what would your energy like to create?*

14 Finish with discussion of the experience of the exercise and the imagined creative expression.

Active meditation

Slow-motion for self-awareness

Age range: 10 years to adult.

The aim of this exercise is to work with focused attention, to connect with the body and let it loosen, relax and to connect with the energy inside. There are lots of directions in this exercise and it may seem very controlled. If children get into a muddle acknowledge this, allow humour. Invite them to relax and take some full breaths and then continue. Soft flowing music will help (see Appendix 3).

1 Begin with simple centring as children stand in a relaxed way with eyes closed. Invite them to bring awareness to their belly for a few minutes.

2 Neck: *Let your neck relax, allow your chin to move slowly down towards your chest. Do it very slowly, feeling each degree of 'letting-go'. Be in the muscles. Include continual letting-go in the whole body and sighing out of 'old' air. Let your neck move slowly all the way down and then up so it is tilting back.*

3 Arms: *Slowly raise your arms up in front of you until they are about level with shoulders, then slowly let go. Keep wrists loose. Feel the use of tension as they rise and the degrees of letting-go as they flow down again.*

4 Knees: *Slowly bend your knees. Keep some awareness in the centre of you. Feel the 'letting-go' as the body goes down and the adding on of strength as you rise up. Keep the rest of the body more or less straight but not rigid!*

5 Arms and knees: *Let arms and knees move together now. The arms rise as the knees bend down. Each time you come up feel the tall point. Keep allowing breath to release. Keep it slow.*

6 Wrists and palms: *Allow arms to flow by themselves. Then add tension slowly through the hands as arms go down. Bend hands back at the wrists. As arms rise wrists are loose; as arms let go wrists are tensed. This tension is felt through the palms of the hands.*

7 Arms, wrists and knees: *Let arms, wrists and knees flow together. There is no 'right' way; you cannot make a mistake. If you get confused simply begin again with just the arms, then add the other parts.*

8 Arms, wrists, knees, neck: *Continue, then add the neck if possible. The neck goes down as arms rise. Keep it slow!*

9 *If possible, add a turning of the torso to the side as arms rise, and back to the centre as arms flow down. First to the right, then to the left. If it all goes wrong relax and start again.*

10 *Let the head free and flow into any shapes or directions or movements.*

11 *Come to stillness now and lie down. Feel what it is like inside you.*

12 Follow with discussion, drawing or journal writing to integrate.

Note: For younger children the first five steps may be enough.

Visualisation and movement meditation
The evening horizon

Age range: 7 to 12 years.
This exercise is helpful for children who are agitated or restless. It allows the restlessness to move, in order to make space for stillness.
Have drawing books and crayons ready.
Have rhythmic music for shaking (see Appendix 3, page 154).

1 Ask children to stand with some space around them.

2 *Take some deep breaths. Shake out the things that are locked up inside you.*

3 *Your breath is magic. It helps you change into lots of different things. You are a firecracker. Gunpowder is packed inside. See what happens when you are lit.*
   • *What colours are coming out?*
   • *What movements do the sparks make?*
   • *What sounds does this firecracker make?*

4 *Become the energies, sounds and movements of:*
   • *a moth flying around a light at night*
   • *a garden slug after the rain*
   • *a hummingbird sipping the sweetest nectar*
   • *clouds blowing across the sky.*

5 *Now you are a young fern in a clearing in the bush. There is space around you. A breeze is blowing from all directions: it changes directions. You are flexible. Feel your roots in the earth. Feel your fronds uncurling and reaching up.*

6 *You are now the horizon. There is the most beautiful sunset ever coming down to meet the mountains. Around you birds are becoming quiet, the humans settle down, the world becomes still. You are the colours, you are the gentle light, the country stretching so wide across the horizon.*

7 *Be this for a while. Feel inside yourself and ask: How do I feel inside? Is it peaceful? Colourful? What is it like?*

8 Ask children to draw the colours and shapes of the horizon.

9 Invite children to tell the group about the main feeling inside them that emerged from the exercise and show their drawings if they wish.

Visualisation and movement meditation

Exploring the seeds of life found in darkness

(from Mary Martin)

Age range: 10 to 14 years.
Have drawing books and crayons ready.

1   *Lie on the floor. Let your eyes close. You are the dark earth. There is nothing to fear. You are peaceful and inviting. You are not static. Feel the sensations in your body of being the dark soil of the earth. Are you heavy, thick, soft, light? Move with the sensations you feel.* (Pause)

Allow your movements to slowly transform into silence and stillness. Gentle, deep breathing. You are the still, welcoming, dark soil of the earth. Bring attention to your breathing now ... the rhythmic movement of breathing in and out. Inhale ... exhale ... one whole breath ... being at one with the breath. (Short pause)

Staying deeply within yourself, turn on your side then very slowly come to a standing position. (Short pause)

You are now a very special seed. You have been blown by a gentle breeze and you are floating through the air and you will soon come to rest gently on the top of the welcoming dark soil of the earth. As you float you are aware of your heart-centre—that place where your deepest longings and dreams reside as well as your true feelings and dark secrets. All of life with its changing seasons passes through your heart—springtime's birthing, summertime's flowering, autumn time's maturing and wintertime's gestating darkness. All of these are in your heart. Allow your heart to go through all of these. At this time, which space is your heart passing through? Allow the feeling of the season of your heart-centre to come to you as you float down and settle on the earth. (Pause)

You are sinking down into the earth now. Let your body move. Down, down, deeper and deeper, into the ground, below the surface, into the darkness. of the soil. Move with this. You are not afraid. There is mystery and wonderment in the dark, quiet depths of the soil. The darkness is not negative or disturbing. It is creative and beckoning. (Pause)

You are a unique seed here in the earth. Become aware of your colour and shape. You lie there motionless, seemingly lifeless. But you know that you are in the womb-like process of becoming. You are aware again of the season that is passing through your heart. You are not worried about this season because you know that other seasons will naturally follow. (Pause)

You are now feeling the refreshing moisture touch you. Allow yourself to welcome the moisture. The darkness around you seems darker with the moisture, but you welcome it all. Maybe you are a little puzzled by it all, but you are willing to be there. You are aware of your heart-centre and its potential. (Pause)

The warmth of the sun is reaching you through the dark soil. You welcome its nurture. You are aware that something is moving deep inside you. Your heart-centre is expanding. Your insides are stretching like you could never have imagined. Allow your body to move and stretch, slowly. (Pause)

Suddenly you break out of the seed. You are beginning to move upwards towards light. Allow the movements to change as you move towards the light. (Pause)

You now come up through the earth, a seed no more. You have pushed your head up above the soil. You are sitting or kneeling up now. (Pause)

The shoot has become a plant now rising up towards the sun. Is the same season still passing through your heart or has it changed? (Pause)

You are a full plant now, green and beautiful, and you are gently swaying in the breeze. Now, out of your heart comes a bud, and the bud gently opens into a wonderful and beautiful flower. Move and breathe as it opens and you become aware of its shape and colour. You are admired by people and insects and animals. You are extremely relaxed with yourself and at one with all that is around you. Out of that relaxation your own special sound or song emerges. Allow that sound or humming to come now. It may be a gentle sound or a very strong sound. Just allow whatever wants to come. (Pause)

2 *When you are ready go and draw whatever aspects of your seed journey you wish.*

3 *Share your drawing with a partner.*

4 *Talk about which part of the meditation you liked the best.*

Walking meditations

Walking, which most of us do every day, can also be a meditation. It does not sound very glamorous or exciting, but older children can develop an almost scientific interest in the mechanics of bringing together awareness and the physical movement of walking. Some Buddhist monks work at it for years, and films of them in practice show the great subtlety of their steps. Their tradition obviously encouraged inner focus, with the movements of the feet as an anchor for the attention.

Most of us actually cling to the earth as we walk, with great tension in our ankles. Our thoughts are usually elsewhere—running ahead to new plans or reviewing the past. We usually miss the beauty of what is in front of us.

75

There are benefits from arousing curiosity about what is possible with inner awareness. Also, a sense of balance and 'at homeness' results from these efforts. It is helpful to advise participants to drop the thinking about the exercise, and to try to drop doing it with mental direction and relax into a more organic body connection. It is good to try these exercises indoors first where there are usually fewer distractions before trying them outdoors.

Here are a few ideas or 'tasks' for turning walking—which you have to do every day—into an activity that will also encourage further inner exploration. The Earthing exercises (see page 90) will be useful as preparation. Walking meditations are essentially earthing work while in action. Presenters could spend time exploring these eight exercises before introducing them to children.

Walking meditations

Age range: 12 years to adult.

Walking meditation
Relaxed walking

1 *Go for a quick walk and observe—from the inside—how much tension there is in your ankles.*
2 *Now try to walk and relax your ankles at the same time.*

Walking meditation
Wandering

1 *Go for a walk just for the sake of inner observation, of increasing your bodily self-awareness.*
2 *Do not think about where you are going. Go with no need to arrive.*
3 *Remind yourself every few minutes why you are taking the walk.*
4 *Notice the tug for your attention from the outside. Keep making the effort to be self-aware.*

Walking meditation
Contact with the earth

1 *Watch where you are going as you take a walk.*
2 *Now turn your attention to the movement of each foot.*
3 *Feel the heel-sole-toe movement.*
4 *Divide your attention. Let some part of your attention stay with the movement and contact in your feet.*

Walking meditation
Slow-motion walking

1 *Try walking very slowly.*
2 *Feel each nuance of change in the muscles of your legs, ankles and feet.*
3 *Sense the changes in your balance.*
4 *What is really involved in walking?*
5 *See what happens if your mind gets active and tries to do the walking!*

Walking meditation
Barefoot in the park

1 *Find a place where it is safe to walk barefoot.*
2 *Focus interest on the textures of:*
   * *gravel*
   * *grass*
   * *cement*
   * *bare earth*
   * *bitumen.*
3 *Notice also the temperature differences as you walk in the shade and the sunshine.*

Walking meditation
Warriors' walk

1 *Walk with your inner awareness turned to your 'hara', the energy centre just below your navel.*
2 *Let breath and energy flow right down into you.*
3 *Keep returning your inner connection to this power centre.*
4 *What do you learn about your habits of being distracted?*
5 *Feel what happens to your energy.*

Walking meditation
I've got rhythm

Part one

1 *Tune into the rhythm of your steps as you walk.*

2 *See if you can synchronise your breath with your steps in some way.*

3 *Enjoy the rhythm.*

Part two

4 *Use the rhythm of your walking to remind you to send your inner awareness into the limbs of your body. For example:*

- *four beats or steps while you focus on the sensation in one leg*
- *then four beats or steps while you focus on the other leg*
- *then four beats or steps for each arm, etc.*

Walking meditation
Zen walking

1 *Sit still for 10 to 15 minutes, focusing awareness within (see Earthing exercises, page 90).*

2 *Before you stand up, try some slow movements while staying connected to the sensation of your body.*

3 *Stand up slowly.*

4 *Now go for a short walk, and keep the inner awareness.*

5 *Come back to your sitting place and ponder on what you have learnt.*

All these ideas provide exercises for 'being at home' in yourself as you go shopping, walking to the post-box, bushwalking etc. When you are more at home within yourself you are able to take in the beauty around you, meet others more deeply, and find a new pleasure in yourself. This personal preparation is essential before guiding others.

We find that these walking exercises, along with many of the others, can begin subtle philosophical questions in adolescents. They can begin to think and ask about the relationship of consciousness to the physical body, the nature of awareness, the meaning of the inner world. Presenters do not have to have answers for these questions. Some educators believe it is best to support them in refining and respecting the process of questioning. The source of creative imagination can be touched into by this questioning.

Active meditation

Basic walking meditation

Age range: 10 years to adult.
This meditation is aimed at supporting the creation of calmness and body awareness.
Give directions slowly; allow time for participants to try each instruction.

1 Ask the group to walk slowly around the room, all in the same direction, in silence.
2 *Begin to feel the floor under your feet.*
3 *Relax your whole body:*
   - *drop tension in neck*
   - *allow shoulders to drop*
   - *let yourself take and release full breaths*
   - *let your belly be soft.*
4 *Be aware of knees. How are they? Tight? Relaxed?*
5 *Now slow down the walking.*
6 *Take three large breaths and let them relax out.*
7 *Become aware of your feet. Feel how your toes, soles and heels touch the floor.*
8 *Try to walk and relax your ankles at the same time.*
9 *Practise walking and feeling your feet from the inside for a while.*
10 Ask children to follow you outside.

Note: You can decide whether the conditions make it suitable for bare feet. If they are, choose a path which provides different textures for the feet to experience.

11 Draw children's attention to differences in:
   - texture
   - temperature
   - hardness/softness.
12 Remind children to bring their attention back inside themselves to feel their feet.
13 Come to a quiet place and ask the group to stop, close their eyes for a moment and feel the earth under their feet.
14 Either come back inside or stay outside and discuss:
   - what it felt like to walk this way
   - how attention is drawn to the outside so easily
   - how the children feel after this exercise.

CHAPTER SIX

Journey to the centre of the Earth

To sit perfectly still and surrender oneself
completely to stillness, whether of the body
or the mind gives the divine element in us
time to become a reality.

Karlfried Graf von Durckheim, *The Japanese Cult of
Tranquillity*

Quiet meditations

This chapter explores preparation for meditation, quiet sitting meditation, evoking the witness state and earthing exercises. It is a time for dropping thoughts about external events and connecting with the sensations and energies in your body. This focus creates a doorway into the source of creativity within. These types of exercises are presented to assist children to move towards the possibility of being still and silent for a while. This stillness, when not forced, can be very calming and healing. Sometimes the word 'centring' is used to describe this quiet tuning-in, especially if the inner focus has been directed to a specific place inside, for example, to what is often called the heart centre (chest) or hara centre (belly).

This focusing allows a reconnection, or deeper connection, to the source of creativity and imagination. Sometimes imagination is used—especially for younger children—to visualise a still, quiet environment that will assist in the creation of a still and quiet inner world for them. With regular, repeated practice this effort can lead to a state of inspiration, intellectual clarity and emotional balance.

Presenters and children should be warned about expecting results too soon. Focus on outcomes or expected changes is actually an interruption to the inner effort. Initial efforts might show, at first, how difficult it is to be focused. Certainly hyperactive children or those with scattered attention or short attention spans will have the most difficulty with this work at the beginning.

There are some recent approaches to personal growth and self-esteem work that try to graft on wonderful experiences or wonderful ways of thinking positively through affirmations. This is not the focus here.

Try to avoid giving too much input or setting up expectations of specific outcomes. Allow children the time, space and support to find their own positive attitudes, that may have been forgotten in the rush of daily life.

Quiet inner focus is an adventure. Although it sounds simple—even boring to some—the effort contains many elements of the mythological hero's journey. There is the leaving behind of a known place, venturing into new territory, confronting opposition, being transformed or growing up in some way, and then the return. It is in the return phase that you can see evidence of the value of inner-life skills approaches. There is value in the calmer attitudes, the gentle excitement about their inner world, the relaxed flow in body movement and particularly in positive behavioural changes.

The range of exercises and experience covered by the word 'meditation', as it is used in various traditions, is too wide to fully explore in this book. There are hundreds of schools of meditation in many cultures. Most focus on one aspect of the process; for example there are yoga schools that affect the inner energy through body postures. There are ways that are designed to influence the heart, the emotions. There are ways that prescribe mental exercises.

Some of the ancient practices of silent sitting—for hours—do not seem to address the modern person's deep tensions and agitation, and are well beyond the needs and interests of children and adolescents. Introduce quiet sitting work gradually, beginning with short times. Make it an experiment and invite students to share their observations of what happened, what was difficult, what helped them with their focused awareness.

Inner focus is about being a witness to the inner world. It requires unprejudiced observation. It involves a choiceless awareness that helps you come into stillness, into an alive, poised state. On the way to this stillness you need to allow deep letting-go of tension, of expectations, analysis and any forcing.

For upper primary and secondary students, regular efforts with quiet inner focus are essential to experience creative results. You may begin with some movement work, then use visualisation stories to set a mood. Sometimes soft music will assist the relaxation and inward focus. Guidance from you to support children to stay with the effort of inward focus may need to be continuous at first. With experience children will be able to extend their inner focus without your constant directions and reminders.

In our culture most of our education, our learning about ways of being in the world, revolve around outer knowledge and intellectual accumulation. The work offered here turns us in another direction, towards learning from inner experience and becoming open, 'empty' and intellectually quiet for a while.

Primary school children could begin with three or four minutes a day of silent, still work. We have seen this comfortably expand to fifteen minutes over a period of several months. To see a whole class sitting silent and still, with eyes closed, and to see the completion drawings and hear the integration discussions is very inspiring. A new, encouraging appreciation of children's developing values will emerge for presenters. Children grow in self-awareness, there is a more positive group cohesion and a new ability to talk about problems and gain support to find solutions. Self-esteem is enhanced as negative beliefs have less hold over children.

Presenter's preparation exercise

First questions to ponder and journal

Read these questions slowly, one at a time, then close your eyes, relax, and ponder for a moment. Then write down your thoughts or answers.

1 *What do you hope to achieve through quiet inner focus?*

2 *What is your own main obstacle to becoming quiet?*

3 *What is the main thing you would like to change in yourself?*

4 *What feels just right?*

5 *In what part of you is your energy most alive right now?*

6 *Do you ever get to an inner stillness or silence? If so, what do you do in that silence?*

7 *What has helped you most in making contact with your inner world?*

When your writing is complete, put it away, and review it the next day. Give your comments, insights and ideas time to percolate, evolve, clarify.

Preparation

Most of us could admit that really we are just beginning to prepare ourselves for quiet inner focus. Most of us know that the calmness that remaining quiet can sometimes bring only lasts a short while. We need to give ourselves lots of experiences of preparing for this: of getting our bodies, hearts and minds to be more willing.

1 Recognise and accept the frequent times of resistance, when the outer world, and our thoughts about it, seem much more interesting.

2 Recognise that inner focus can lead into either:
  • more stillness
  • the awareness of tensions and unsettled emotions.

3 Connect with your body through:
  • relaxation and surrender, consciously using tension, then letting go
  • movement, shaking and vibration, walking briskly, dancing
  • massage
  • sound as a way to release tension, for example, singing, humming, shouting
  • using music to help tune in
  • taking time in a hot bath to relax the body
  • quiet times in nature to 'listen' within.

4 Emotional release. Do you need to unload emotional stresses?

5 Become aware of your breath. As an ongoing practice become more aware of when it feels free or restricted.

Most of our initial work before quiet sitting will be clearing our 'chaos', letting old suppressions be thrown out. This is preparation for being truly still and awake. Buddhists practise to remove the five 'hindrances'—sensual passion, ill-will, sloth, worry and perplexity—from the mind before quiet inner focus. Inner-life skills work with children and adolescents often needs to address the same hindrances.

Practical preparation of the meditation space is essential. Firm cushions that allow the hips to be raised slightly higher than the knees are ideal. A carpeted floor will make ankles more comfortable when sitting cross-legged and for times of lying down in deep relaxation. A quiet space, with outside distractions reduced, is ideal. Obviously presenters should try out these exercises at home. Taking the phone off the hook and asking family not to interrupt will be essential.

Some basic stages

There are several stages in the work of meditation. Knowing these stages will support programming the exercises progressively. From familiarity with these stages you can create new formats that can really meet children 'where they are'. The time each child takes to progress through these steps will be different. Some may need to stay with steps 1, 2 and 3 for a long time, even several months; others may be ready to proceed within a few weeks. All this depends on the group attitude, the confidence of the presenter, the attention spans of the children, their clear motivation for doing the work, their age and readiness to participate, etc.

The usual stages in quiet sitting work are:

1 Moving and freeing the body, dealing with agitation.

2 Coming home with stillness. Beginning to 'anchor' awareness in the body and letting go of wandering thoughts, relaxing the body.

3 Staying with an active effort to pay attention within. This may involve outer direction and reminders.

4 Allowing deeper relaxation. Letting effort become 'non-effort'. Becoming more receptive to subtle sensations and energies within. Constantly letting go of the inner story about what is happening in order to sense a more direct experience.

5 Allowing breath to relax and become gentle.

6 Entering the witness state, a state of 'creative emptiness'. Witnessing the experience. Allowing and feeling the flow of new energy and creativity while in this state.

7 Emergence of subtle positive feelings resulting from new harmony and new energy. This is often felt as pleasure and peace.

8 Re-entering the outer world without immediately abandoning the inner world; staying connected within.

9 Finding positive ways to express the creative energy, for example, through drawing, projects and hobbies.

Meditation exercise

Following the basic stages

Age range: 10 years to adult.
Have firm cushions ready for sitting meditation.
Have drawing books and materials ready.
Give instructions slowly; some may be repeated. Leave a pause between each set.

1 *Run on the spot for a minute. Shake. Talk out loud about all the things that are bugging you right now; say it to the wall in nonsense language.*

2 *Now sit down on your cushion. Cross your legs in a way that is comfortable.*

3 *Close your eyes and feel your breath coming and going. Can you feel your heart beating after that running?*

4 *Let your mind focus on feeling what is happening in your body now. Let your body be soft and relaxed.*

5 *Our main effort in the meditation is to keep coming back to the world inside you. It is as if you are on a safari through your inner land, watching the scenery, watching for any animals. You must try to stay alert. There are two things that will help:*
   • *feeling your breath come and go*
   • *feeling your body and the energy inside it.*
   I will remind you to bring your attention back to these.

6 *Now allow a deeper relaxation:*
   • *let your neck relax and go a little bit soft at the back*
   • *let your shoulders drop*
   • *allow a fuller breath now*
   • *make sure your belly is not held tight*
   • *let your legs and feet be soft now.*

7 *Let your breathing relax. Don't try to do anything with your breath.*

8 *You are simply watching the inner world now:*
   • *What are the sensations in your body?*
   • *What are the main thoughts or pictures in your mind?*
   • *What are you feeling?*
   Simply be aware of all this.

9 *Watch inside for any peaceful feelings or happy energy.*

10 Now slowly and gently move your toes and fingers a little. Let your limbs stretch a bit, and when you are ready let your eyes open. Try to stay in touch with your inner world as you look out at the outer world again. Don't talk to anyone yet.

11 Take some time to draw how you feel now, to draw any special pictures that came into your mind while we were sitting still. We can talk about the exercise soon.

Evoking the witness state

The witness state is a delicate balance of attention where you are able to watch what is happening in your inner world without interference. This state helps us dis-identify with the contents of consciousness, and simply become more conscious. It is a state that most of us can reach only after considerable practice. It is a state that is the aim of many ancient traditions. It may be achieved more easily by older children with clearer motivation.

Experiences of this subtle state will give children a feeling of freedom and centredness—a state from which important decisions can be made or new directions for life can be recognised.

The next exercise gives some hints for beginning to work towards this state. These hints could be given to a class of older students—in suitable language—as they begin to attempt quiet inner focus on a regular basis.

Meditation exercise

Guiding students towards the witness state

Age range: 15 years to adult.

(Pause between each step.)

1 Ask students to sit in an upright yet relaxed position.

2 *Remind yourself why you are making this effort to achieve quiet inner focus. Remember there are benefits from feeling calmer and happier such as relating to others in a more positive way. This effort with inner-life skills will strengthen your ability to concentrate on the work you have to do.*

3 *Is there any resistance? Are there parts of you that don't want to do it? Quietly recognise any parts like this.*

4 *Be aware now of your posture. Can you make it balanced, naturally stable, with the least possible tension?*

5 *Let your eyes remain closed or gently fixed in one direction. If you are more comfortable with them open let them be unfocused, and try not to look around the room.*

6 *Tune in to your breath now. Allow it to be soft, even, relaxed. Never force it.*

7 *Surrender is the ideal state to begin from. What does this mean to you right now? Is your body surrendered? Is your mind relaxed and surrendered? It is important to simply acknowledge if you do not feel surrender at the beginning.*

8 *Nothing dramatic is expected in this meditation work. There is no one to prescribe your experience. There is no right or wrong. You cannot fail.*

9 *Any struggle shows that you have not dropped down into the witness state yet. How can you allow any struggle or strain to dissolve away? Let your effort be one of focused attention and surrender.*

10 *Do you notice any expectations in yourself? Expectations begin in our mind. They take us away from the inner-world experience of each moment.*

11 *As you sit here quietly you will get used to finding yourself lost in thoughts of the future and memories of the past. Practise self-acceptance. Notice that you have been 'lost' and then simply return to your work with the meditation. Waste no energy on self-criticism.*

12 *Open to a state of witnessing, of being in contact with what is happening inside in body, mind and feelings. Try to witness without commentary. Aim to let go of the mind's way of trying to tell us everything all the time.*

13 *When you find a quiet witnessing state—even if just for one second— be glad of it. See if you can stay still and quiet for a little longer.*

Quiet inner focus exercise

Watching the candle flame

(From Patricia Nolan)

Age range: 6 to 12 years.
Have a small birthday cake candle, holder and matches ready.
Quiet, gentle, flowing background music may be useful for children who are not used to silence.

1 *In a little while I am going to light this small candle. All the time it is burning, I want you to watch the candle and breathe deep breaths, in and out. While you are watching the candle, you can make any sounds you want and any movements you want, or be still if you like. Just keep breathing fully all the time the candle is burning and let yourself relax. You can blink as much as you need to, but try not to look around the room too much. When the candle goes out you can lie down. When you lie down you can have your eyes open or closed, and just enjoy whatever the feeling is inside, and rest.*

2 Ask children to gather sitting in a circle, about 2 or 3 metres from the candle.

3 Set the candle in a holder, slightly raised, so that the children's line of sight is slightly upward. With beginners, cut a little off the candle. Experiment beforehand to get a length of candle that burns for about 2 to 3 minutes at first.

4 Light the candle, and play soft music in the background.

5 Tell children to breathe fully.

6 When the candle has burnt out completely, invite children to sit or lie down for a few moments with eyes open or closed, letting the body rest.

7 After a brief rest time invite them to draw how they feel and/or discuss the experience.

Quiet inner focus exercise

Heart centre awareness

(From Paul Perfrement)

Age range: 10 years to adult.

Have quiet, settling music in background and encourage an open, relaxed, trusting posture, preferably with children lying on their backs, arms by their sides and palms facing upwards.

1 Ask children to lie down, relax and get comfortable with eyes closed.

2 Read the directions slowly, pausing between areas of inner focus. Guide children to slowly scan through the body from feet up to head.

   Become aware of your feet, the lower half of legs, the upper half of legs. Bring your awareness to your pelvis and lower back, then to your abdomen, upper back and chest. Relax again and tune in to your shoulders and arms, your wrists, hands and fingertips. Now move your inner focus to your face, neck and head. (Allow at least 4 minutes)

   Note: If children need further relaxation repeat this step, adding the act of tensing the area of the body then relaxing and exhaling.

3 *Focus on the movement of breath in your belly, chest, throat or nose.* (Allow about 3 minutes)

4 *As you continue to focus on the breath, see if you can drop thoughts as they arise. Every time you notice that you are thinking, simply let the thoughts go and return to the awareness of the breathing in your body.* (Allow about 3 minutes)

5 Guide participants to become aware of the centre of their chest. Continue to use the movement of the breath as anchors for their awareness.

   Each in-breath now expresses all that you long for in life. Picture the things you long for as you breathe in and feel them in your heart.

   Each out-breath represents letting go and surrender of everything. With each breath let go of any worries, tensions, thoughts or negative feelings. (Allow about 6 to 7 minutes) (Pause)

6 Occasionally remind them to let go of thoughts, return to breath awareness and the intention at the heart centre.

7 Quietly ask children to 'come back into the room' by:
   • connecting with their breath
   • feeling their body on the floor
   • moving their hands and feet gently
   • opening eyes.

8 *Share your experience of the exercise with a partner. Talk about the three main things you experienced.*

Variation: Those with more experience of meditation might include, during an extended quiet time, the use of a repeated word (mantra), for example, love, life, I am. The mantra is gently sounded on the in- or out-breath, can help relaxation and centring and serves as a means of connecting within more deeply.

Earthing exercises

Each of these morning meditations begins with children sitting in a balanced posture—ideally sitting cross-legged, with the hips higher than the knees. However, sitting upright in a chair will do. Take time to allow the body to settle and the mind to disengage from the previous activities. The aim of these exercises is to begin again and again, rather than struggle to stay focused. Do not make a problem out of distraction. Practise letting go of distractions and beginning the exercise again.

Presenters will need a high level of patience and acceptance of children's ability and willingness to participate, as well as their own ability to work with inner focus. Discuss frankly with children your own efforts in order to support an atmosphere of exploration and discovery together. Emphasise that the work is not about attainment and 'getting it right'.

The exercises can help loosen control of endlessly revolving automatic thoughts and allow more attentiveness to gather. This effort will be supportive of other learning tasks. They allow for subtle relaxation in the body. These formats have been gathered from many traditions, and have been integrated into modern stress management and relaxation training. Some have also begun to appear in courses for busy business executives, to help them manage stress and to increase their access to spontaneous new (and profitable) creative ideas.

These earthing exercises are built around the basic stages of quiet inner focus (see page 84). They present simple ways for older children to work with focusing attention on body sensation in order to quieten wandering thoughts. The ordering and structure of the areas to be focused on also helps focus the mind, and shows up more quickly where the revolving thoughts have played their tricks of distraction.

Earthing exercise

At home in my hands

Age range: 8 years to adult.
Have a tennis ball, apple or orange for each child.
Have quiet music in the background, with a slow, even rhythm.

1 Ask children to sit comfortably, in a way that allows their breath to be full and their energy to flow up and down the spine. Their left hand should be resting on their knee and the right hand turned up holding the ball (or fruit). The inner eye, the inner focus, is on the right hand, feeling the weight of the ball.

2 Encourage children to allow breath to be full, and to feel the sensations of the hand, feel it supporting the ball; feel what is inside the hand, feel the air on the skin, feel the texture of the ball.

3 Tell them thoughts, ideas, distractions will come, but the inner work is to keep coming back to the focus on their hand, to let their thoughts float away.

4 After a few minutes ask children to change the ball to the left hand and refocus on the left hand.

Note: If the attention span is short, keep changing the hand for focus.

5 After about 3 minutes for each hand (for children over 13 years make it a little longer) ask children to place the ball on the floor in front of them and then continue as if they were still holding it, imagining its weight and shape, and continuing to focus attention on the hands.

6 After a few minutes invite them to shift their focus into the middle of the body and continue the effort of sensing what is there.

7 End with a simple question such as: *What is it like to be at home, inside yourself?*

8 Ask children to respond to the question in words, writing or with drawing.

9 Conclude with a group discussion on their experience.

Note: There is benefit in repeating this exercise on a regular basis.

Earthing exercise
Coming home

Age range: 12 years to adult.

1 Ask children to sit cross-legged on cushions or in a relaxed and balanced posture in chairs, ideally with eyes closed.

2 *Bring the attention to the right hand, simply waiting until there is some inner contact with how it feels inside.*

3 *Is it warm? Is there any feeling of buzzing or tingling in it? Does it want to move about?*

4 *Now move your attention slowly around the limbs as I direct you, in this order: right hand, right arm, right foot, right leg, left foot, left leg, left hand, left arm.*

5 *Allow your attention to remain in each part for a few minutes, opening to really connect with the sensations.*

6 *What is the temperature of the air on your skin? Can you feel the places where your hands or feet touch your clothing or the floor? Can you feel the warmth inside your hands? Can you feel the vibration of energy?*

7 *Let's begin again and go around the body, moving your attention as if it was a torch shining on the inside of each part.* (Continue as in Step 4.)

Earthing exercise
Breath and energy flow through all of me

Age range: 14 years to adult.

This exercise is based on the idea that the air we breathe contains energy. This energy can be more consciously taken into the body.

While we sit quietly, our attention follows the breath, and the energy that comes in with the breath, down through the body on the out-breath. Attention moves, flows slowly from the chest (lungs) down through the torso to toes and along the arms to the fingers. On the in-breath the attention returns to the chest. Presenters simply guide the movement of attention and remind children to constantly return within.

Earthing exercise
The two main centres

Age range: 12 years to adult.

1 Ask children to sit cross-legged on cushions or in a relaxed and balanced posture in chairs, ideally with eyes closed.

2 Focus all your attention on your chest. Tune in there for a moment. Feel it rise and fall. (Pause)

3 *Now move your attention down to your belly, see if you can feel it from the inside, let it relax and hang loose.*

4 *Now move your attention to your chest on the in-breath, then drop it down to focus on the belly during the out-breath.*

5 *Your attention will simply fall and rise between the heart area and the belly area, along with the breathing.*

6 *Your breathing should remain natural and relaxed.*

7 *We will work this way for a while, feeling first our chest from the inside, then our belly.*

8 *There is nothing else to do. Simply stay quietly focused inside yourself.* (Pause)

9 *Every time a new thought comes into your mind, and you realise it has taken your attention away from the exercise, sigh out all your breath as if you were sighing out the thoughts that get in the way. Then begin again.*

10 *In these exercises we begin again and again.*

Earthing exercise
Only breath

Age range: 14 years to adult.

This approach uses the breathing as the focus for attention, without any interference. Children simply use the natural movement that accompanies breathing as the anchor for awareness, returning to sense this movement over and over. The temperature and pressure of the air as it moves in and out of the body is noticed. There are very subtle sensations that are possible to perceive. This subtle attentiveness brings forth a state of calmness, and enlarges the arena of consciousness. It is important to avoid *doing* anything with the breath in this exercise, as this encourages the ego. Of course doing something is more satisfying to the ego!

Encourage children to give this exercise a 'fair go', perhaps trying it at least three times before deciding if it has any effect.

Earthing exercise
Navel gazing

Age range: 14 years to adult.

The term 'navel gazing' is linked with the Eastern tradition of focusing awareness in the belly. Simple hara awareness is based on deciding to use one centre as the inner focus, and returning to it over and over. 'Hara' is the Japanese name, in Zen, for the energy centre just below the belly button. Inner focus on the area forms one of the main efforts of quiet Zen sitting.

This exercise is deceptively simple. It consists of sitting, with closed eyes, or gently unfocused eyes, and turning all the attention within the belly. The belly is relaxed, and children simply try to keep their attention in the belly, returning there every time a distraction is recognised.

For the ego that likes a challenge, this exercise may seem too simple, but if we watch what happens we will usually connect with a rampant, scattered attention that could benefit from some taming. Allow 5 minutes for primary children at first, then increase to 10, and eventually to 15 minutes at a sitting. The length of time can be increased gradually as children feel ready and have some experience of the benefit of the resulting balanced inner state.

Earthing exercise
Return from the source

Age range: 14 years to adult.

1 Children begin by imagining the centre of the body—like a line or tube running down through the centre. Awareness is then focused at the centre of the body, at the core. Children spend some time focusing in the centre.
2 Then gradually the attention is moved slowly out to the skin.
3 After some time of being aware of the skin, the attention is guided back inside to the centre.
4 This movement of attention from the inner core to the skin is repeated several times.

Earthing exercise

Journey to the centre of the Earth

Age range: 14 years to adult.
Before beginning the exercise discuss the idea that we have an energy core, deep in the centre of the body. This core has been described in Eastern literature. Sometimes it is seen as a fire, sometimes a gentle energy flow up and down the body. Children can be invited to sense what it feels like to them.

The focus within begins with awareness on the skin—sensation of air, touch of clothes, etc. Awareness then moves gradually inwards towards the core. Children need to take time to sense energy at the core of themselves. This slow movement of attention is repeated over and over, as if allowing the body to become permeable to energy, light, life. This inner focus work is attempted for a short time—about 5 minutes—at first. Older children may wish to progress to 10 or 15 minutes.

Earthing exercise

Attention dissolving tension

Age range: 14 years to adult.
This exercise uses Wilhelm Reich's division of the body into seven segments that work together to hold or release emotion and energy. These segments have functional contact and relate to the seven chakras of the Eastern traditions.

1 Ask children to sit cross-legged on cushions or in a relaxed and balanced posture in chairs, ideally with eyes closed.
2 Children allow attention to connect then move down through each segment (the segments are listed below) of the body. They begin at the crown of the head and wait with focus there until there is a connection with the sensation. As the attention drops down to the next segment physical relaxation should follow. This relaxation will probably be very subtle and may be accompanied by a natural sighing out of breath.
3 The sequence should be:
   * crown
   * ocular segment—eyes, ears, back of skull
   * oral segment—jaw
   * cervical segment—neck (especially allow surrender at the back)
   * thoracic segment—shoulders, chest and arms
   * diaphragmatic segment
   * abdominal segment—belly and lower back
   * pelvic segment—pelvis, buttocks, legs and feet.
4 Repeat the exercise two or three times and end with awareness in the whole body.

Earthing exercise

Welcoming energy pathways

Age range: 17 years to adult.

1 Ask children to sit cross-legged on cushions or in a relaxed and balanced posture in chairs, ideally with eyes closed.

2 Children allow attention to move slowly up the back on the in-breath, beginning at the sacrum and rising up to the crown. On the out-breath the attention simply flows down the front—from the crown to the lower belly.

3 Ask children to visualise the energy moving in this circle. After about 7 to 10 minutes the attention rests in the whole body.

Earthing exercise

I live in a seven-storey building

Age range: 10 years to adult.
The speed of presentation can be determined by the attention span of the children. The exercise is designed to begin to bring awareness to the seven areas, traditionally associated with the body's energy centres or chakras.

1 Ask children to sit cross-legged on cushions or in a relaxed and balanced posture in chairs, ideally with eyes closed.

2 *Picture yourself as a tall building with seven storeys. You can move around inside yourself. Through the middle is a lift. It can stop at each floor. There are different things happening on each floor.*

3 *Mostly you live on the sixth floor. It is the one with big glass windows, and you can look out to see all the business around you. This apartment is in your head!*

4 *Actually you have been living up here so long you have forgotten what is on the other floors! So today you will go down and up to check out what is on the other floors. So, take a look around this apartment on the sixth floor. What is here? Thoughts? Bits and pieces of today, this morning, things from yesterday? It is usually cluttered with things.*

5 *Now imagine you are moving to the centre of the main room. There is a round lift. Get your torch and step in. Press the button marked 5. The door slides closed. You go down.*

6 *The door opens. There is a dark room. This is inside your neck, your throat area. This is the room where sounds are made. Take a look around. Do you need the 'torch'?*

7 Guide the children through visits to the other floors, asking them what they 'see' inside. Colours? Pictures? Type of room?

4th floor: chest/heart

3rd: middle of body/diaphragm area

2nd: belly

1st: hips/legs

The 7th floor, the rooftop garden, is the top of head and is the last floor visited.

8 Ask the children to draw an outline of the building then add colours, pictures and symbols of what they found at each floor. Younger children may need to draw their outline at the beginning of the exercise and colour in their responses between the visits to each floor.

9 Complete the exercise by asking children to write a general summary statement of the main things going on in the building.

10 Discuss these summary statements.

CHAPTER SEVEN

Cultivating creative seeds

We must try to understand the symbolic
language with which the many-sided
psyche expresses itself in images and
dreams. Thus, we can reach the psyche's
creative seeds which are able to effect a
transformation and change in a child's
relationship to life.

Dora Kalff, *Sandplay*

A language for the inner world

Symbols and imagery are often called the language of the imagination. The individual imagination is an expression of the unconscious. Artists, designers, composers and scientists—in fact all who make creative leaps in their work—use their imagination. Each psyche has a creative potential. The exercises in this section are designed to help children tap into that creative potential. They also support children to take the images or fragments of fantasies that may contain rich expressions of their inner world seriously. Taking the inner world seriously also supports self-esteem. The work with visualisations can generate enthusiasm for creative writing, artwork, drama and personal development.

In inner-life skills work symbols provide an extended language for understanding and expressing subtle experiences, sensations, emotions, realisations. Symbols and imagery are fluid, expansive and not limited by set rational meanings as words so often are.

Many children—and adults—are greatly helped to recognise their inner world through symbols. They feel safe to acknowledge the symbol, and gradually become more directly aware of what is being symbolised. In some cases the unconscious will present low self-esteem, pain and upsetting emotional memories in a symbolic form at first. This prepares children to remember and feel directly, so that healing can take place.

Just as a toddler feels relief when language becomes effective, children experience satisfaction and fulfilment when subtle areas of their inner world find new ways to be recognised and communicated. Using symbols and imagery is a good way to begin this process of recognition and communication of the strengths, feelings, ideas and directions that in many children remain out of sight, ignored in favour of the academic curriculum.

We all have an in-built mechanism that directs our psyche towards wholeness. In order to be re-owned, the disconnected parts of our psyche, of our character, often appear as symbols in dreams, in fantasies and in visualisation work. The symbols can represent positive aspects such as talents, courage, the ability to care or emotions seeking release. Pondering the meaning of a symbol—even imagining ourselves becoming a symbol through role-play—that has been presented from within, can help reconnect with the inner world.

Direct symbol interpretation by another person is not useful for children. They need to feel and understand the meanings within themselves. Many positive or spiritual symbols are presented to children from their unconscious when there is a need to counter-balance negative experiences in their outer lives. Positive symbols can be easily remembered and, when explored, can become a force that supports self-esteem.

Symbols that are important for children can appear during visualisations. You can use the visualisations in this book or use them as a guide for creating your own. Older children love making them up! After the story stage, guide children in acknowledging their special Self through drawing, discussing, role-play and writing about the symbols that the unconscious presents during a visualisation exercise.

Since the symbols presented by the imagination hold an energy in the unconscious, the role-play is important to allow that energy to express itself and thus be made available for daily living. (See Appendix 1, page 150.)

Visualisation

Visualisation work is focused, active use of the imagination. It can be directed, given boundaries, or free form. Most visualisations lead children on a journey that brings them to a threshold, an imaginary or real place that becomes familiar in the exercise. It is usually a natural, safe, beautiful place and is used as a doorway into the realm of their own imagination. The journey part of visualisations prepares a clear space in their mind for the imagination to reveal its contents.

Asking them to use their own imagination, you can direct children to explore beyond the threshold of the given story. This prepares a space for their own symbols, imagery and story to emerge. Then they are guided to return to the starting point, bringing something new with them.

Visualisations work well both with groups and individually. They help children awaken to positive feelings about themselves. It may be very supportive for younger children to invite them to describe the discoveries, as they find them, to a partner who simply listens. This helps them stay in touch with the imaginary journey. Sometimes they could be drawing during the visualisation, but usually lying down with eyes closed assists them to enter it more deeply. Quiet music can be used to set the mood.

Stages in threshold journey visualisations

1 An overview of the exercise and reasons for doing it.

2 Relaxation work, centring, body awareness.

3 Visualising a safe, beautiful setting, involving the senses in the descriptions.

4 Describing the threshold that the exercise has led to, for example, a gate, a clearing in the forest.

5 Allowing the imagination to present its own symbols, images and story.

6 Returning to the threshold.

7 Visualising the journey back to the starting point, retracing steps.

8 Returning to outer reality.

9 Recording symbols, images, gifts, words of wisdom, etc.

100

10 Communicating through discussion about the experience.

11 Exploring any relevance of the images to children's daily life.

Visualisation often uses images from children's sandplay, dreams, favourite fairy tales and universal symbols, including the energy of popular heroes/heroines from film and television. Visualisations, as part of the inner-life skills work, explore themes of discovery of inner treasure and inner strength, inner stillness, resolution of conflicts, and often set the scene for inner guidance and clarity. This guidance comes from a level of the psyche deeper than the rational—but often chaotic—mind.

The study of drawings created after visualisation journeys will reveal much of what is happening in children's inner worlds. These can help you trace the development of self-awareness, self-esteem and the success of increased access to the imaginative realm. Over time, a series of these drawings can be used as part of your evaluation process.

For very active or disturbed children, exercises that alternate tensing and relaxing the body, such as bioenergetics (see pages 64 and 65), will be a necessary preliminary to being able to be still enough to close their eyes and allow inner focus.

Visualisation exercise

A gift for now

(from Dorothy Bottrell)

Age range: 10 years to adult.
Have crayons, drawing books and journals ready.
Have gentle music in the background.

1 Ask children to sit or lie comfortably, with eyes closed, and follow the directions.

2 *Be aware of how you are breathing. Now allow yourself to take three deep breaths and let yourself relax as you breathe out. Feel yourself relaxing more with each breath. Notice how it feels inside and let your whole body relax.*

3 *See yourself standing at a gateway. There are two large gates. Look around and see where you are and notice the details of the gates.*

4 *The gates are opening now and you walk through into a huge garden. It is very lush and green.*

5 *There is a path. Follow it and notice how tall the trees are, how beautiful the flowers are. Look at their colours. Stop and smell their fragrances. What a beautiful place!*

6 *Continue along the path. Enjoy this place, enjoy being alone, just you amidst all this lushness!*

7 *The garden now opens out into a large area of lawn. You walk barefoot across the cool grass. Imagine the softness of the grass under your feet.*

8 *Finally you come to some sand which is beside the ocean. Feel the sand between your toes. Feel the dampness and firmness of it as you walk closer to the water's edge.*

9 *See the huge expanse of ocean, listen to the sounds of the waves crashing. Look around and take in the beauty of this place.*

10 *Smell the salt in the air. Feel the warmth of the sun on your back, across your shoulders, warming your whole body.*

11 *Feel the freedom of this place.*

12 *Now it is time to return. Take a last look at the ocean, then walk back over the sand and onto the grass. Feel the change in texture under your feet again. The sounds of the ocean become fainter as you walk back towards the gardens.*

13 *Follow the path back through the trees. As you walk towards the gates you notice someone standing there. As you get closer you recognise her or him. The person looks like you, but older. That person is your future self, the person you will become.*

14 *Notice what the person is wearing. How does he or she look?*

15 *What qualities does he or she seem to have?*

16 *This person has something to give you. It is a special gift from the future to bring back with you now. Accept the gift. Thank the person.*

17 *Now walk on back through the gates.*

18 *Now start to come back to this place here now (at school, in this room, etc.) Feel yourself sitting (or lying) comfortably. Feel what is under you.*

19 *When you are ready open your eyes.*

20 Encourage children to stay connected to their own thoughts and feelings as they draw the gift that they received.

21 Give children several questions to write about:
  • *What was the gift and what does it mean to you?*
  • *Describe your older self. What are your responses to this image of who you may become? For example, Does it feel right? Does it surprise you? How does this image make you feel?*

Visualisation exercise for finding personal symbols
The wisdom of the landscape within
(From Paul Perfrement)

Age range: 14 years to adult.
Have relaxation music ready.
Have journals ready.

Part one: The journey

1 Ask children to select partners for the second part of the exercise.

2 Ask children to lie on a carpeted floor on their backs, in a relaxed open posture with eyes closed.

3 Guide children through a relaxation, including breath awareness and awareness of feelings and sensations. (See Meditation exercise on page 85.)

4 Begin the visualisation journey. Elaborate on:
   • a journey in a canoe, paddling down a stream
   or
   • a walk in a meadow or forest.

5 Encourage children to observe the imagery, to allow it to do whatever it does, and learn from it.

6 After a while, suggest to children that they interact with whatever it is that catches their attention in their imagery. If they don't have any imagery at this point suggest they go back to whatever stood out or was significant for them earlier.

7 Invite children to ask the image that has stood out:
   • *what it has to tell them*
   • *what it needs from them*
   • *whether it will help them in some way.*
   Children let the energy of the image accompany them to the next stage.

8 Invite children now to focus on their belly, to experience the feelings that are there.

9 They allow a new image, a word or symbol to emerge while they focus on their belly. This could be an animal, a person, flower, star, rock, etc.

10 Allow children some time to interact with this symbol. Encourage their focus to stay with the symbol. Children ask their symbol:
   • *what it has to tell them*
   • *whether there is anything it needs*
   • *if there is anything they can do for it.*

11 Encourage children to imagine themselves providing or receiving this information or help immediately.

12 After a minute or two, children move their focus to the throat area and repeat the steps above, opening to a symbol.

Part two: Integration

13 Direct children to spend time linking their inner experience with their life now.

14 Children record what happened in the belly and throat areas, and what they saw.

15 They reflect on and write about how this relates to any present experience in their lives and how what they experienced could help them in some area of life.

16 Children form a large circle with the whole group, each person standing beside her or his partner. Ask children to face out from the centre.

17 They focus within again and reconnect with their main symbol—the one that seemed most important to them.

18 With some deep breaths they open to letting the energy of the symbol be in their body now: they role-play the symbol.

19 As the symbol they take on a posture that helps them feel more like the symbol. Then they move as it would move and make its sound.

20 They turn to their partner, and take turns at saying:
  • *I am ...* (symbol)
  • *I look like ...*
  • *My main purpose is ...*
  • *I have a message for ...* (own name). *It is ...*

Note: Details for this stage are discussed in Appendix 1, page 150.

21 Allow time for feedback in a discussion with the whole group.

Visualisation exercise

The gift from a wise part of me

(From Elysha Neylan)

Age range: 10 to 14 years.
This exercise is ideal for completion of a period of group work.

Part one: The special place

1 After some dancing or movement, ask children to sit or lie down and close their eyes.

2 *You are going on an adventure. Imagine it, see it in your mind. You are walking along a path to a very special, sacred place. What is it like on this path? How does it feel not knowing about the place you are going to?*

3 *You are coming towards the end of the path now. You can begin to see the special place. You are moving closer to it. See it more clearly now.*

4 *It could be familiar to you or a place you have never seen before. See what is there, see the surroundings. Is it near the beach? In the forest? In the outback, the desert? A rainforest? On a mountain? Let your mind imagine the place.*

5 *It is a very safe place, a place that makes you happy to be there. Find a spot to sit in this place. This will be your own special spot.*

6 *Now in this place lives a very wise person. In your mind, look up and see this wise person nearby. This wise person will be your friend.*

7 *Look carefully. What does this wise person look like? What is this person wearing? How does it feel to be with him or her? Is he or she near to you now? Or far off? Sitting? Standing? Moving?*

8 *You didn't know this when you set out on this journey, but there is a gift here for you, in this special place. The wise person knows what it is. It is not a gift like a toy or a camera. It is a gift you feel inside you, like happiness, excitement: something you like to have. It might be a new feeling you have never had before.*

9 *Listen to the wise person. You will be told about the gift and be helped to receive it. This special place can let the gift just slip right inside you very easily. You are surprised to learn that part of the gift is that you will become the wise person of the special place now! Feel yourself changing into the wise person.*

Part two: The celebration

10 *Now let yourself slowly stand up. See if you can keep your eyes closed for a little longer.* (Play gentle rhythmic music in background.)

11 *Let yourself dance as this wise person and feel the gift inside you.*

12 *Now let the gift of the good feeling spread out inside you as you dance.*

Part three: A symbol in the stillness

13 *Now be very still for a moment. Take some full breaths.*

14 *Stay connected with the gift inside. Imagine what this feeling would look like if you could photograph it. (Alternatively: Go to the sandplay shelf and find a symbol that reminds you of your gift.)*

15 *Draw the symbol or show it, then share the meaning of the symbol. In what way is it like the inner gift, like the wise person? What is the symbol reminding you about?*

Note: If working in groups, make a group picture of the drawings or symbols or explore making a group sandplay.

Visualisation exercise

Feeling my strength

(From Patricia Nolan)

Age range: 10 to 14 years.
This exercise is especially useful for children who are feeling overwhelmed or vulnerable to outside forces. It allows children to connect to inner strength.

1 *Stand with your eyes closed.*

2 *Feel your feet firmly on the floor. Close your eyes if you are comfortable doing it. Take a few deep breaths and relax them out.*

3 *Picture this. Your energy passes through the floor down into the earth beneath. Imagine feeling the soil on your feet, really feeling the touch of the soil, the cool, brown earth against the soles of your feet.*

4 *Now imagine there are tiny little roots growing out of the bottom of your feet reaching down towards the earth. Going deeper into the earth. Becoming thicker now ... much thicker ... very big thick roots ... getting stronger now ... very strong, deep roots ... big thick strong roots ... going right down deeply into the earth.*

5 *These roots are your roots ... growing out of you ... so strong and deep ... growing so deeply into the earth ... holding you to the earth.*

6 *A strong wind begins to blow. Feel it moving through your branches, bending your limbs, making you sway a bit this way and that. Feel how your strong roots hold you steady even though the wind tries to blow you over.*

7 *You are a tree in a valley. Now there's a flood coming down the valley. Feel the torrents of water rushing into your trunk, trying to*

uproot you. Feel how your strong roots hold you firmly to the earth.

8 *Now a bushfire is coming, burning your lower branches, burning and singeing your bark. It feels like it's going to burn you right up, but it doesn't. Rain falls and puts the fire out and there you are still standing deeply rooted.*

9 *You are firmly in your place. Breathe into that strength, your solidness, your connectedness to the earth.*

10 *Draw a picture of yourself as the strong tree. For example, draw yourself with the strong roots going down right through your feet.*

(Pause while they draw)

11 *Talk about how you feel:*
- *What happens in your life that you need these strong roots for?*
- *When you go home how could you help yourself when it feels like there are no strong roots?*

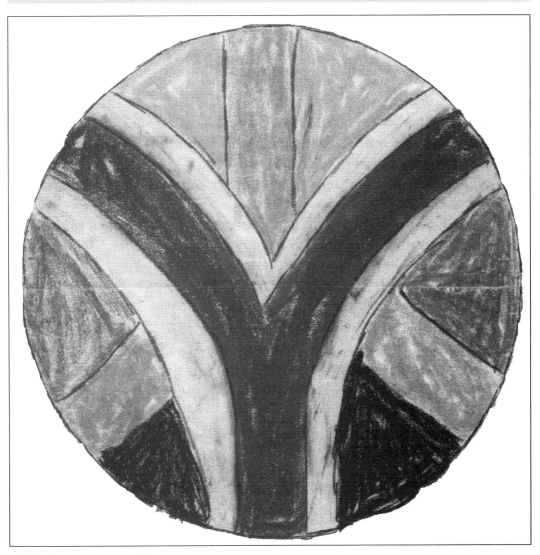

'This is my strength'
Mandala by a 10-year-old boy, after the exercise 'Feeling my strength'

Visualisation exercise

The tribal island

Age range: 10 years to adult.
Have drawing books and crayons ready.
Have a copy of the Gestalt role-play question sheet (see page 150) ready for each pair.

1 Ask children to select partners for the second part of the exercise.

2 *Imagine yourself as part of a tribe that lives beside the ocean. Stand up and take some deep breaths. Feel your feet firmly on the floor.*

3 *You are dancing around the fire with your tribe. You dance on into the night. It is a full moon. The moon is shining a silver path out across the ocean. The water is calm. The night is warm. Something is calling you to take your canoe and venture across the water.*

4 *You paddle out, following the moon's path. You paddle and paddle, but you don't get tired.*

5 *The daylight glows orange and yellow on the horizon. You see an island. You know that is your destination.*

6 *You paddle ashore to the island.*

7 *On the shore you walk up the beach. Feel the sand.*

8 *You head into the middle of the island through the trees or jungle. There is a track that guides you.*

9 *You come to the entrance of a clearing. You see there is a clearing in the middle of the island.*

   Note: Give children time to imagine going into the centre of the clearing to discover what is there.

10 *In the centre of the island will be a surprise, something wonderful and unexpected. Watch and discover what is happening there. Watch and see every detail.* (Pause)

11 *The day gets hotter. You must return now to your tribe.*

12 Guide children back, stage by stage, from the clearing, across the ocean, to their own land and tribe.

13 Children report to the chief of their tribe, and draw what they saw in the clearing on the island.

14 Ask children to role-play what they found in the clearing in pairs. (See page 150 for the Gestalt role-play question sheet.)

15 Ask each child to discuss the message of her or his surprising symbol, and any relevance it might have to her or his daily life.

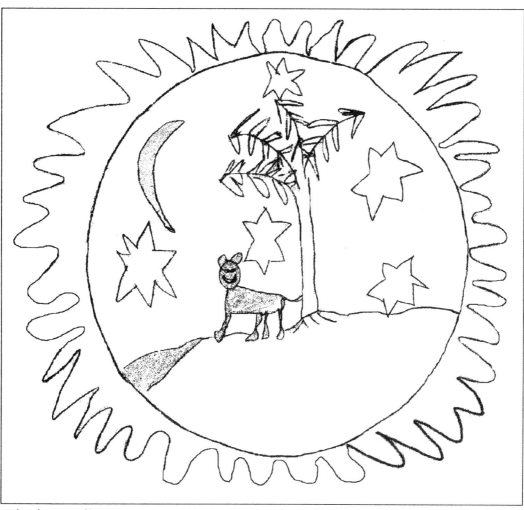

'The happy lion'
Drawn by an 8-year-old girl, after the exercise 'The tribal island'

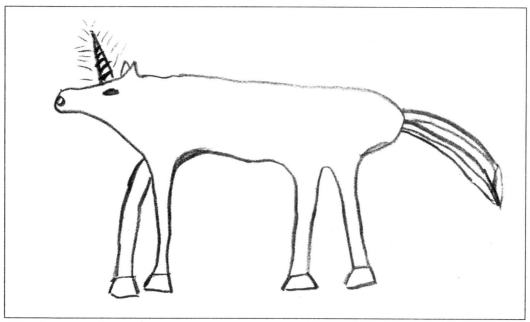

'The brave unicorn'
Drawn by an 8-year-old girl, after the exercise 'The tribal island'

Visualisation exercise

Earth people

(From Patricia Nolan)

Age range: 10 to 16 years.

1 Ask children to sit in a circle.

2 *Take some deep breaths, all the way down to your tummy.*

3 *Close your eyes.*

4 *Imagine now you are part of a special people on the earth: the first tribe. There is something special you have come here for.*

5 *See yourself as part of this earth tribe. You can be big or small, you can be any colour you want to be.*

6 *Your home is deep down in a cave. See the cave. Feel what it is like in this cave, your home.*

7 *You have come to this place where you are now going to experience something special.*

8 *There is something special in the air. Imagine what this specialness looks like. Is it like magic? Does it have a colour? Does it have a shape? Let yourself see it in your mind.*

9 *Breathe it into you.*

10 *With this specialness inside you, part of you now, you can know what the special reason is you have come here for. It might come into your mind as a picture, or a memory, or an idea. Wait for it.*

11 *When you have a feeling of what you have come here for, draw a picture.*

12 When all the children have finished drawing ask them to hold up the pictures to the group. Ask them to think about, then speak one sentence about their specialness.

Visualisation exercise

My hero/my heroine

Age range: 10 to 16 years.

This exercise can be used as a focus for a directed visualisation involving older children's favourite heroes or heroines. This will embody some aspect of their inner life (or missing inner life). It is ideal for small groups.

1 Guide children into relaxation and quietness.

2 Invite them to let a picture come to their mind of a hero or heroine that they admire. It could be someone from real life, or a character from film or television.

3 Ask children to take the hero or heroine to a dangerous, exciting or mysterious place in their imagination.

4 Invite them to 'see' the place clearly.

5 Tell the children a story will unfold as they watch. In this story the heroine or hero will be confronted with some difficulty.

6 Leave some minutes for the children to discover the story and for the hero or heroine to confront the difficulty.

7 After some minutes, guide the children through their return journey.

8 Ask children to develop a short play—with others—and act the part of the hero or heroine. Ideally all children should have the opportunity to act out their play.

Visualisation exercise using imagery for relaxation
A storm at sea

Age range: 8 years to adult.
This exercise invites reflection and then harnesses agitation and conflict. By acknowledging it and then allowing it to resolve through imagery, children can move into a calmer state. This exercise is helpful for children who are in emotional turmoil. They realise that storms do end, and peace can follow.
Have drawing books and materials ready.

1 Ask children to sit or lie down.

2 Describe the scene of a storm at sea, and ask children to see it in their mind as you speak:
   - *turbulent waves, thunder, lightning, coldness, waves breaking against ships, deep waters rolling and heaving*
   - *the sea and the weather gradually quietening and becoming still*
   - *the waves settling, becoming a simple rise and fall like the children's breath*
   - *the clouds part, the sun comes out.*

3 Ask the children to wait and see what happens now. What comes across/over/from beneath the water?

4 Leave time for the children to imagine the next scene.

5 Ask them to draw what they saw.

6 Discuss how it would feel to be in the storm. Ask them to consider if there is anything in their life that is like this storm, or if they sometimes feel like a storm themselves.

Note: Children with very active energy may benefit from acting out the scene.

Visualisation exercise using imagery for relaxation

The wild hurricane

Age range: 8 to 14 years.
This exercise is a visualisation about power, choice and gentleness. It shows that very active energy can be guided and transformed.

1 Ask children to stand with space around them so they can move with the story if they wish. It is best to close eyes, unless children are making large movements.

2 *Imagine you are a hurricane, travelling across the land, furiously. A hurricane is a huge storm with violent, fast winds.*

3 *You pick up everything in your way, whirling it around and carrying it off.*

4 *You spin everything all around, uproot trees, take roofs off houses.*

5 *Do you want to throw it all in the sea? Into outer space? Dump it back on the land?*

6 *No. Today you decide to put it all back again, just how it was.*

7 *Picture yourself as a slower wind now, gently dropping everything back in its right place.*

8 *You've become a gentle breeze. The clouds are gone and the sun is shining. The birds are singing—they are not afraid now.*

9 *How does that feel?* (Students lie down or sit now, becoming still)

10 *What's happening now? Watch inside and see.*

11 Give children time for the imagination to yield what is needed.

12 Invite children to draw the part of the story they liked best.

13 Follow drawing with discussion.

Symbol exercise for pondering problems
Pictures of my life on a rock

Age range: 12 years to adult.
Presenters can learn a great deal about a particular child from working one-to-one with this exercise.

1 Children choose a partner and decide who will go first. One will listen while the other explores the exercise. Then they will swap roles.

2 Everyone walks in the garden, or in the bush, for about 5 minutes, in silence.

3 *Look for a rock that attracts you. It needs to be one you can hold in your hand. Note its place carefully so that you can put it back exactly where you found it.*

4 *When you both have a rock, sit down together. The one who is exploring first closes eyes and thinks for a moment about the main problem or difficulty in his or her life.*

5 *When you are ready open your eyes and begin looking on one side of the rock.*

6 *On the rock, as you look patiently, you will see some shapes emerge. Keep looking until you can see a picture of something natural like a tree or an animal. (Pause)*

7 *Tell what you see to your partner.*

8 *The partner who is the listener says: 'How is it connected to your problem?' and nothing else. You do not discuss it. Your partner will help you remember the pictures.*

9 *Take a moment to feel what the rock is saying with this picture, what advice it is giving you. Talk about this. What other way of looking at your question or your life is it presenting? (Pause)*

10 *Turn the rock to the next side and continue in the same way until you have looked at it from four different angles and found pictures.*

11 *Then share with your partner what all four pictures told you, going back to the first angle, then the second, and so on.*

12 *When you have finished, you thank the rock and put it back where you found it.*

13 *Now swap roles and begin to listen to your partner. I will guide you through the same steps.*

14 Invite children to draw pictures of the images they saw on the rock faces.

15 To support integration, ask children to record their insights or messages in their journal.

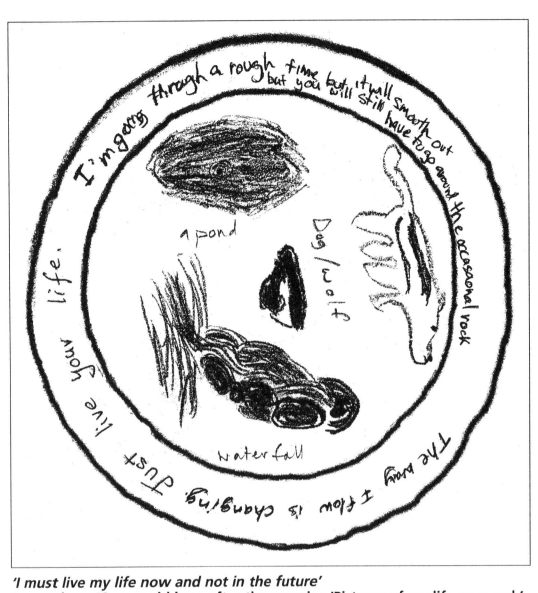

The writing around the rock reads: "I'm going through a rough time but it'll all smooth out but you will still have to go around the occasional rock. The way I flow is changing. Just live your life."

Labels inside: a pond, Dog/wolf, waterfall

'I must live my life now and not in the future'
Drawn by a 13-year-old boy, after the exercise 'Pictures of my life on a rock'

CHAPTER EIGHT

Reclaiming a lost world

When I see a child in therapy, I have the
opportunity to give her self back to her, for
in a sense a poor self-concept is a lost sense
of self. I have a chance to bring her in
touch with her own potency, to help her
feel at home in the world.

Violet Oaklander, *Windows to our Children*

Focus on self-esteem: developing hope and inner strength

The exercises presented in this chapter are particularly aimed at supporting an increase in self-esteem. They also support children's ability to articulate about their inner world, and about feelings, hopes and aspirations—all of which are vital to healthy development. They are particularly useful for integration after emotional release work.

Through self-discovery, self-esteem can be achieved using inner-life skills. Visualisations and Gestalt exercises are used to help children recognise their own value. It is best to avoid creating any dependence on external valuing for self-worth. Inner-life skills use imagery and play to bring forward children's forgotten positive qualities.

Enhancing children's positive sense of self is the combined task of parents, teachers, carers, counsellors and grandparents. Violet Oaklander, in *Windows To Our Children* (1988), lists several basic guidelines for every-day relating that will support self-esteem:

- listen to, acknowledge and accept children's feelings

- treat them with respect

- give specific praise

- be specific in criticism—don't say 'You always ...'

- be honest with them

- own your reactions to children, don't blame them

- give responsibilities, independence and freedom to make choices

- involve them in problem-solving

- be a good model—think well of yourself.

When children have missed out on this regular supportive relationship there is a need for both emotional healing—release work—and reconnection to the original positive self-relationship. As Oaklander says: 'All babies think they are wonderful'.

Affirmations and goal setting are often considered useful approaches to personal growth and helping children attain self-esteem. It may certainly be true that positive thinking has a beneficial effect, but be cautious about artificially glossing over inner turmoil and lack of self-esteem with wonderful affirmations, given by others.

Clinical observations of ERC have shown that thought has no lasting power over emotions. If it did we would all be well controlled and children would not repeat the outbursts that so often get them into trouble. An affirmation may make a child feel good for the moments he or she is thinking of it, but unless it has organically grown out of inner work, come from the child's inner world, it really has no lasting impact.

Many presenters and counsellors teach affirmations to children. But who has formulated the affirmation? Is it a product of a hopeful ego? Is it someone else's suggestion? Has the child tried to perceive the parent or teacher's expectations?

It is more helpful for the healing process to bring forth positive attitudes in children from which to set goals rather than to have them make lists and promises. Younger children may need help in finding the right words for their own positive statements about themselves—experienced during an inner-life skill exercise.

To find this place within they will need quiet inner focus and possibly some emotional release work. Much lack of worth is connected with an overload of held-in emotions and self-blame. If you find that the exercises here are not sufficient to bring forth a child's positivity about himself or herself, it may mean that the child has old emotional obstacles that need to be healed in the unconscious. Working with this may need the support of a counsellor who is confident in emotional release.

Feeling good about ourselves through achieving outer goals set by another person is not therapeutic. It does not bring deep healing. It can, in fact, reinforce the imprint that 'I am no good as I am', 'I have to achieve in order to have value'. It is a superficial 'feeling good', and not helpful for long-term balanced development. Try to avoid cheering children up through proving that they can achieve. Listen carefully to any of their self-doubts and criticisms. Make sure they know you are really listening and can hear their pain.

It is vital that goals, wishes, intents, steps, new directions are indeed set by the maturing part of children, found through their inner world. It is also vital to eventually discover—and this is in the realm of counselling—the source of negative or limited beliefs and self-images. Knowing that negative self-images have been taken in from the outside is a major step in separating from them. It may be the first time children realise that what they thought were facts are really just beliefs.

Many of the children and adolescents we have worked with have had little to look forward to emotionally. The exercises here helped them to find again the hope, the creativity and inspiration that had been buried inside.

The exercises in this chapter all use imagery. Many include role-play of positive images to help children re-own positive qualities within themselves. This method of role-play has been developed from Fritz Perls' dreamwork method (*Gestalt Therapy Verbatim*, 1969).

Writing down and speaking out positive feelings about themselves is a most important step for children. This often goes against the grain for the Australian character, where to appreciate yourself can bring condemnation. It will be helpful to ritualise, and even formalise, the time when children share with others the positive messages that have come from their work with the exercises. Really being heard by others helps them to hear the positive messages themselves. It challenges the old way of being.

Self-esteem exercise

My reflected beauty

Age range: 8 years to adult.

This exercise is most successful when there is a beautiful view, a wide outlook across a valley or river or a colourful garden. It is particularly useful for children or adults who believe an old imprint about themselves which reinforces their low self-esteem.

Have drawing books and crayons ready.

1 *Choose partners for the Gestalt role-play part of the exercise.*

2 *Go outside with drawing paper and crayons. Look around in all directions. Look up and down and around. Take some quiet, deep breaths. Notice everything you can about the scenery. Wait for a few minutes and feel yourself as part of this scene. Observe what nature is showing you.*

3 *What stands out as the most beautiful, the most wonderful? What is the part of the scenery that you like best? Take some time to look carefully around. Something will stand out for you as the most beautiful.*

4 *When you find it, draw it carefully. Then come back into the room to work on the next part of the exercise.*

5 Ask children to role-play, in pairs, what they have drawn, following directions from the Gestalt role-play question sheet (see page 150).

6 Invite children to show their drawings to the group and share the message and how they felt about the message.

Self-esteem exercise

Your magic power animal

Age range: 10 years to adult.

This exercise helps children find supportive strengths deep inside, and to carry an image of the strength as a reminder that they do have resources to cope with their worries.

Have drawing books, or large sheets of paper and crayons ready. Have clapping sticks or rocks ready.

1 Ask children to choose partners that they trust.

2 Invite children to stand in a circle in a large clear room.

3 *All life is a journey. We are all given the strength to face our fears, to face those big problems and worries, and to make our lives wonderful and exciting. But usually this strength is hidden inside us. Today we are going to call it out of hiding. And we need help for this.*

4 *Discuss with your partner the hardest things in your life, the biggest worries or problems, things that you need help with.* (Pause)

5 *We will now go on a journey to find the help we need. The help will come from a magic power animal, a spirit animal. This spirit animal lives on a distant island. This island exists deep in your imagination. Once we get to the island we will need a special chant to call the animal out of its hiding place. Let's practise it now:*
   I am here, waiting alone.
   Come to me, waiting alone.
   Repeat it over and over. Clap the rhythm of the words.

6 *Now we will build a canoe to cross the waters to this island. Build it out of cushions or chairs or beanbags. It must be big enough for everyone.*

7 *Collect your clapping sticks or rocks as you get in the canoe.*

8 *Stop now to take some deep, slow breaths to gather your energy for the journey.* (Pause)

9 *Take up your paddle and paddle together with a steady rhythm.* (Drumbeat)

10 *We row all day. The sun begins to set. We row faster, counting out the rhythm.* (Darken room if possible)

11 *The island is in sight. We come into shallow waters. We stop at the sand. We step out. Look around in your imagination. See the sea, the rocks, the sand, the grass, the trees in your imagination.*

12 *Find your special place to wait for the magic animal. You must go alone—the animal will appear just for you. Imagine the beginning of the sunset. Become quiet and still.*

13 *Your special magical spirit animal is somewhere on this island. It is time to call out for it.*

14 *Using the clapping sticks or rocks, begin the chant.* (Chant as before for a few minutes) *Close your eyes. Keep them closed so that you will see the animal appear in your mind.*

15 *See how the animal appears. Does it swim? Fly? Hop? Run? See it clearly, every detail of its body.*

16 *Now it comes close to you. It wants to talk, but you cannot understand its language. But this is a magic animal, a special magic spirit animal, so it makes you into its twin.*

17 *Feel yourself becoming the same as this magic animal. Move a bit, make its sounds. Feel your fur, or feathers, or fins. Feel the animal's special strength.*

18 *Listen to it talking to you. Is it giving you a special message, or passing on to you its strength?* (Pause)

19 *Now it is time to say goodbye to your animal. The moon is coming up in the sky, and we must get back to the mainland before morning.*

20 *See your animal go. As it goes you become a person on the outside, but inside you keep the feeling of that strength.*

21 *Go back to the canoe, sit down in it next to your partner.*

22 *Row home together, quickly now with all this new strength. We row on past bedtime, past adults' bedtime, past midnight. The sun begins to rise.* (Lighten room)

23 *Now we arrive safely at the shore.*

24 *Get your drawing things and draw your animal. Draw it very carefully so you won't forget it.* (Proceed after they have drawn pictures)

25 *Share with your partner all the qualities of the animal that you like. Share how your life would be, how any big problem you had would be, if you always had this animal strength.*

26 Ask children to gather again in a large circle to show the drawings.

27 With everyone clapping a rhythm, ask each child in turn to come into the middle and dance and make the sound of her or his animal.

Visualisation exercise for self-worth

Inside the spaceship

(from Margaret Thomson)

Age range: 9 to 13 years.

This exercise helps children connect with inner knowing, to be more confident of listening to inner wisdom.

1 Ask children to lie on the floor and get comfortable. Take some time to allow them to relax.

2 Ask them to take big breaths in and sigh them out.

3 *I want you to imagine you are moving along a path. This path leads you into a very bushy forest. You feel very safe as you are wearing a very special watch. This watch warns you if there is any danger around you.*

4 *As you push past a big bushy tree you come upon a clear area. You stop. Right in front of you is a spaceship landing in the middle of the clearing. As you watch, the door opens and some travellers from another planet come marching out and disappear into the bush.*

5 *You have a chance to explore the spaceship now. You set your special watch on safety alert, knowing it will warn you if there is any danger. You carefully move towards the spaceship, up the steps, through the door, into a winding corridor.*

6 *As you move slowly along inside the spaceship, you become aware that the floor slopes down and around. And you keep following it. You pass a door. You have a peek in. It's not the main room so you keep going further down and around. You check your trusty watch, it has never let you down.*

7 *You move along further. There is a door into a room in the very middle of the spaceship. You go into this room. It is like a movie theatre with seats and a special screen.*

8 *You sit on a seat and the screen lights up. It says special messages just for you. You watch and some cartoon-type characters come on the screen.*

9 *They talk to you and call you by your name. They tell you something very secret and special about yourself. Take some time to listen to what they are saying.* (Pause)

10 *When they are finished you thank them. You stand up and the screen goes blank. You move back to the door and along the corridor.*

11 *As you move along you are aware of the slope of the corridor going up, up and around. You come to the doorway and peek out into the daylight. It is all safe.*

12 *You run down the steps and into the trees. You wait, hidden behind the trees. The space travellers come back. The spaceship*

takes off. You go back on to the path that led you to this place. You follow it back.

13 *Soon you find yourself coming back into this room.*

14 *Feel your feet and toes, feel your fingers. Stretch a little.*

15 *When you are ready, gently open your eyes.*

16 Ask children to do a drawing of what they imagined, and write down their special message.

17 Lead children in a discussion about the place inside them that always has this special information.

Visualisation exercise for self-worth

The special message

(from Margaret Thomson)

Age range: 9 to 13 years.

This exercise aims to support children to focus within for centring and finding peace and calmness.

Have drawing books and materials ready.

1 Ask children to lie on a carpeted floor on their backs with hands and feet uncrossed and eyes closed.

2 Ask children to take a few deep breaths.

3 *Imagine you are breathing out all the tension in your body. Take another deep breath—exhale with a sigh. Take another big breath and exhale. Let your body go soft now.*

4 *Imagine you are walking in your favourite place on this earth. Is it a rainforest? A beach? A flower garden? Is it under the sea? Where is your favourite place?*

5 *Imagine you are in your favourite place now. You are the only one to know about this place. It is your special place. You take some time looking all around you.*

6 *You notice there is an opening, like a door on the far side of this place. It might seem strange to have a door in this place. Take a good look at it now. It has a lock with a key in it.*

7 *You go to the door and unlock it. You see a long corridor on the other side. There are more doors on either side of the corridor. Some are large, some are small, there are many shapes.*

8 *As you look ahead down the corridor, you see a door at the end. You walk towards the end door. As you get close you can see your name on the door.*

9 *Then you see a key and you take the key, unlock the door and go inside.*

10 *You find yourself in a room. Is it big or small? See what picture comes into your mind.*

11 *You are alone in this room. What colour are the walls? The ceiling? Notice the feeling in this room. How do you feel while you are in this room?*

12 *There is a special message for you in this room. It has been left for you by the wisest person on Earth. It is something important for you. The message may be written on the walls, you may hear it spoken out loud, or it might come in a feeling. Take some time to hear or see or feel your message. Remember it. (Pause)*

13 *When you are ready, imagine you are starting to walk towards the door. Open the door and go into the corridor. Close your special door and lock it with the special key.*

14 *Now move down the corridor and back to your sanctuary. Moving back through your favourite place on this earth. Coming back, coming back to this room.*

15 *Feel your toes and hands. Open your eyes when you are ready.*

16 Support children to tell or write the message.

17 Invite them to draw a picture of the room and/or the favourite place.

Visualisation exercise for self-worth

Meeting your inner wisdom

Age range: 10 years to adult.

This is an exercise to give confidence and trust in inner knowing. The sharing stage needs careful attention from presenters.

1 *Lie down, relax, let the earth support you. Breathe—let it out, sink down, there is just now.*

2 *Imagine yourself in a very safe place. Let the image come to you. Are you in the open air? In a room? See every detail. You are feeling safe, comfortable, warm, relaxed in this place.*

3 *Now you see the wisest person on earth. He or she is coming into this safe place with you.*

4 *Notice:*
   - *if this person is male or female*
   - *if this person is old or young*
   - *any special details*
   - *the person's clothes.*

5 *Feel the person's vibes. What can you tell about him or her?*

6 *Now this person offers to be your guide, your mentor or support person. What would be the most important question you would ask?*

7 *See the two of you together. Standing? Sitting? Close? Apart?*

8 *How do you communicate? Speaking? Thoughts only?*

9 *How does the person respond?*

10 *Think again about the question you would like to ask him or her.*

11 *Hear the answer to your important question. (Pause)*

12 *It is time for the person to go. What are her or his last words of advice upon leaving?*

13 *See how he or she leaves now. Watch and wait.*

14 *Now breathe this safe place into you—take it inside. Where in you could this safe place settle?*

15 *Spend some time in silence now. (Pause)*

16 *When you are ready bring your awareness back into this room, gently stretch your body, open your eyes.*

17 Invite children to write down the question they asked and the response.

18 Ask children to draw something to remind them of this safe place and the wise person.

19 In discussion point out that the wise person is in fact really a part of them.

20 Suggest to the children they put the picture up at home and look at it every day for a week.

21 In the discussion direct each child to integrate their experience in this form:
   - *I am ... (become and describe the safe place).*
   - *I am ... (become and describe the wise person).*
   - *I asked ... (say the important question).*
   - *My wise part knows ... (give the answer).*

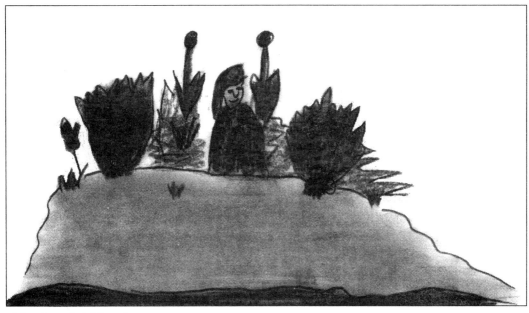

'My Special Place'
Drawn by a 12- year-old boy, after the exercise 'Meeting your inner wisdom'

Visualisation exercise for self-worth

Inside me is the very best

Age range: 9 years to adult.

This visualisation exercise uses Gestalt role-play to explore images that represent the good things of our inner being, our inner resources in symbolic form. These images can represent the light that helps us face the darkness of emotional pain.

Have a page of drawing paper folded in half or quarters, depending on the number of gifts to be explored for each child. Have crayons ready.

1 Ask children to choose partners for the integration part of the exercise.

2 *Lie down and relax. Get comfortable and close your eyes.*

3 *You are very wealthy. Very, very rich. So rich that you could buy absolutely anything you desire. Today you are going to buy gifts for yourself.*

4 *You only like the very best, the most luxurious, the finest quality.*

5 *Sometimes you go shopping with your pockets stuffed with hundred dollar notes, sometimes you just use a special Gold Mastercard, which has no limit.*

6 *You jet around the world seeking out all the very best shops. You have your own jet, of course. See yourself in the jet, sipping some lemonade, issuing orders to the pilot to land in some special country where you wish to go shopping.*

7 *Now you are walking down the street. See the shops, make them up in your mind. You go inside one. What sort of shop is it?*

8 *You are going to buy yourself a very expensive gift. Check that you feel good buying something wonderful for yourself. Select, in your imagination, the biggest, the best, the thing that attracts you the most. Wait, see what that will be.* (Pause)

9 *Draw it.*

10 *Lie down again. Your chauffeur is taking you back to your jet. Off you go to another country. Watch for voices that tell you one thing is enough. Go to another shop, buy another gift for yourself.*

Note: Depending on the age of children and the attention span, they could go shopping to buy two gifts.

11 *Draw again.*

12 *You are going to become each special gift. Each gift represents wonderful qualities in you—get ready to hear about them!*

13 *Sit with your partner now, and take it in turns to tell each other about yourself in the way I explain now.*

14 *Find all the words to describe yourself as you become each gift:*

What you look like, your colour, shape, size, texture, what you are made of.

15 *Say what you are for. Listen to your voice, listen to your words.*

16 *Say what kind of energy you have.*

17 *Share what you have learned about yourself. Remember that each gift is a symbol for some real quality in you that caused you to think it up. The gifts are symbols, the qualities are real!*

18 *Now we will swap and the other partner shares.*

Variation: Older children, after buying the gift could:

- *travel to view an exotic animal in the wild*
- *find the best meal with the food they love most*
- *go to the best concert in the world, the one they would love most to attend.*

Integration exercise

Inside me/outside me

Age range: 9 years to adult.
Have sandplay symbols (or magazines for cutting out).
Have drawing materials ready.
Have a round plate or compass for drawing a large circle.

1 Ask children to draw a large round circle in drawing book.

2 Ask children to choose a partner for sharing about the exercise.

3 Invite children to lie or sit comfortably, close eyes, relax and tune in to their inner world.

4 *Feel what it is like now, what is going on inside you—share this with your partner.* (Pause)

5 *See what pictures come into your mind when you think about the difficult things in your life now. Talk about these.* (Pause)

6 *Find a very special secret part of you that is deep within and describe what it is like.* (Pause)

7 Ask children to find a symbol from the sandplay collection (or cut out a symbol from magazines) that goes with each of the three reflections above.

8 Ask children to arrange these symbols in and around the circles they have drawn and think about how these three things fit together.

They show how these things fit together by the way the symbols are arranged. The arrangement of the symbols can be changed as they share with their partner.

9 Ask children to make up an adventure story with their three symbols as the main characters. They write, tell or draw the story.

Visualisation exercise

The well

(From Pat Quinn)

Age range: 12 years to adult.
Have drawing books, crayons and writing materials ready.
Have quiet music in background.

1 Invite children to lie or sit comfortably, close eyes, relax and tune in to their inner world.

2 *Close your eyes and tune into your body. Take a full breath and relax it out. Allow your body to relax. Come down, out of your head, out of your thoughts.*

3 *Imagine an old-fashioned well that goes deep down into the earth. You are sitting or standing beside it. It is a deep well. The well is in very lush green country and it is full of water.*

4 *You lower a bucket that goes deep down inside the well. It goes down, deeper and deeper.*

5 *This is the well of wisdom—it always gives a message that will help you. It has its own wisdom deep inside—just like you.*

6 *As you wind the bucket up you see there is something in it. It contains a treasure.*

7 *You are now looking clearly through the water in the bucket. The treasure is a symbol or a picture that has meaning for you. Is the treasure floating gently on the water, or resting on the bottom of the bucket?*

8 *Let yourself see it in your mind's eye. Take time for the picture to present itself clearly.*

9 *Whatever you find in the bucket has meaning for your life now. Think about this. Allow yourself to listen inside yourself to receive the message. (Pause)*

10 *When you see or hear it clearly, open your eyes and write about it or draw it. (Pause)*

11 *Think about this message, then share with a partner how it relates to your life now.*

Visualisation exercise for self-worth

Finding my heart

(from Margaret Thomson)

Age range: 6 to 9 years.
Have drawing books and materials ready.

1 Ask children to sit or lie down comfortably with eyes closed.

2 *Take a moment to be still and quiet now. Let your body relax and go floppy. Take two or three big breaths.*

3 *Imagine you are outside, walking down a path. As you go around a bend you come across a beautiful place. This beautiful place is your own special place. Nobody else goes there. Nobody knows about it but you. You stop in this special place and see it clearly in your mind.*

4 *You look around carefully and notice a special old chest. It might look a bit like a pirate's treasure chest. This chest is made from the most beautiful timbers. The hinges and lock are golden. You move closer to it, admiring it.*

5 *You find a key next to it. To your surprise the key has your name on it. You open the chest.*

6 *Inside there is a glowing golden heart-shaped treasure. This treasure belongs only to you. It gives out love.*

7 *You pick up this heart and put it beside your heart. It feels good. It has magic and it helps you find love. You let yourself feel this for a while.* (Pause)

8 *You know now that you can come to this special place, unlock the chest, and use the treasure to feel your own love whenever you want to.*

9 *You put the golden heart-shaped treasure carefully back in the chest and use the key to lock it. You bring the key with you.*

10 *You move slowly away from the chest. You know that you can come to this special place any time you wish. You move back down the path, back to where you started in this room.*

11 *When you are ready, stretch your fingers and toes. Move your body a little. Open your eyes, stretch a bit more if you wish.*

12 *In a moment draw your special place, the chest and the heart-shaped treasure.*

CHAPTER NINE

Attending to each moment of life

From some grand overview of life, it may seem that only the big events are ultimately important. But to the soul, the most minute details and the most ordinary activities, carried out with mindfulness and art, have an effect far beyond their apparent insignificance.

Thomas Moore, *Care of the Soul*

Caring for your inner life

Supporting this personal development work with children, adolescents and adults is a strong belief that the psyche is designed to move naturally towards maturity, health, wholeness. There is a need to release all that stands in the way of wholeness—especially to drop old habits of living with a low level of self-awareness. This chapter aims to help you in your own inner life.

Bringing self-awareness work to children and adolescents assists their intrinsic impulses to explore the inner world. Attempting it yourself activates your own interest in self-discovery. Can you educate yourself in new healthy habits of focused awareness? These healthy habits allow for freer choice in life directions and the smaller daily choices between positive and negative experiences.

What stops you being fully aware of your body now? What stops you being free with the flow of your feelings? What distracts you from knowing your thoughts and at the same time hearing the sounds around, seeing all the sights? These are the sorts of questions we might ask ourselves after beginning work with meditation and relaxation.

Another benefit that comes with meditation is the growth towards more centredness, receptivity, creativity and well-being. This brings greater enjoyment of life.

This chapter explores some traditional possibilities for advanced awareness-in-action work for those preparing to teach meditation. Some of these ideas can be passed on to the young adults and older adolescents with whom you work. They are included primarily as an encouragement for presenters, teachers and youth workers to extend their interest in the inner world and to be more able to inspire students.

When the interest in inner growth takes hold, all the old 'obstacles' become material for the inner work, inner journeying. You might notice tensions, automatic talking, emotional reaction that takes you away from simply being present, focused on what is in front of you. Whatever you find that seems to be between you and your 'presence' can become your particular material to work with, to learn more about during each day. Young people often find that the awareness-in-action work really satisfies and stimulates their emerging philosophical questioning and the awakening of their ideals.

In any moment of the day you can be aware of your energy, your feelings, your thoughts, the sounds around you and the visual impressions. You may notice there is a habit of being distracted by the sound, or lost in emotions, or in what's happening outside. The challenge is to break this habit of being constantly distracted and come back home to yourself. This is advanced awareness in action.

Could the conditions of life, the daily routine, the constant interactions with others be reminders about your wish to return home to yourself? How can you use these conditions to do this? As you work towards greater self-awareness, you receive the energy of life in a more vivid way that brings replenishment of your own energy.

Replenishment of your energy in daily life is supported by an inner-focus practice called expanded or divided attention.

Divided attention calls for part of your awareness to be very present to what you are doing in the outside world and for the other half to be focused on what is happening inside you. The work presented so far—with the exception of the walking exercises—has had an almost total directing of attention within. All this is good preparation for focusing within and without simultaneously.

Dr Alexander Lowen, in *Bioenergetics* (1975), stated that the ability to be clearly focused within and clearly conscious of all that is around us is a sign of bioenergetic health. The more you have established this inner contact in quiet, still times, the more it is possible to divide the attention in the times of outer action.

This consciousness of what is going on inside allows you to use your body wisely. It allows you to make the effort to sense the body, watch the mind and observe the mood—that is, to know yourself, as Plato instructed. This dual awareness is described in many traditions of inner growth.

Divided attention is one of the main inner practices that can transform daily life into a yoga—or Karma Yoga, as it is known to many Asian cultures. This is essentially bringing an advanced effort of awareness, not just in special quiet times, but also during the activities of daily life.

There were, traditionally, several ways or methods of yoga. Hatha Yoga is a yoga focusing on inner work with the body; Bhakti Yoga is a way in which every action is offered as devotion to the divine, thus allowing freedom from the ego's fixation on results.

Karma Yoga, or The Fourth Way as G. I. Gurdjieff and Pytr Ouspensky called it, is a way of being attentive to the whole of yourself while engaged in the requirements of the outer world. The special feature of Karma Yoga is work with focused attention.

There are two types of attention you can have easily. The first type is common: your attention goes where it will, it is *scattered*. If the phone rings your whole attention is attracted to it. Someone may come into the room and you forget what you were talking about because all your attention has gone out to that person. You have a scattered attention that is waiting to be attracted—anywhere! This is most obvious in children who are emotionally disturbed.

The second type of attention begins when you focus on something, for example, something you want to learn—your attention is *directed*. At this moment your attention is primarily directed to these words. Already, directing the attention brings a new level of clarity—you become more aware. This directed attention is what teachers want to develop more fully in children in the usual classroom activities.

There is another type of attention which is a possibility, but does not come automatically, except in very special moments. It involves directing the attention *out* and *in* at the same time.

Visualise an arrow, pointing out as you pay attention to outer impressions. At the level of divided attention the arrow has two heads—one is pointing out, one is pointing in. At first you will have to alternate focusing out, then in. It is possible eventually to be able to receive both outer and inner impressions at the same time. You could be reading, for example, and listening to the resonance of the meaning inside you, feeling the weight of the book in your hand. Open to life outside and life inside. This can double incoming impressions and bring much aliveness.

A person who has developed centredness is capable of this advanced awareness. It is another benefit of inner focus practice, not normally taught in our culture.

There are other levels beyond this, which are possible if you are very alive and have practised for a long time. The next level can be called *free attention*. In this state your attention becomes strong enough to be free, to include effortlessly all that is outside and all that is inside. There is no barrier between inside and outside. But you need to remain wary of dreaming of future possibilities without firm anchoring in the present.

The state of 'sleep', as Gurdjieff calls our normal consciousness, is one in which your attention is scattered, wandering anywhere to whatever is the newest or loudest stimuli. Advanced awareness in action calls you to:

• first, focus your attention; direct it either inwardly—as in quiet inner focus—or outwardly, giving your very best to the work at hand

• secondly, try to keep some attention within yourself (returning to some internal centring, or earthing place) and at the same time send some attention out to be very conscious of what you are doing, where you are; being present to the sounds, the sights, the smells and to the people around you.

This dividing of attention is extremely difficult. It requires a constant wish to see yourself in action, to learn and to grow. It reveals very unflattering aspects of old unconscious habits. This Karma Yoga is a way of inner work within daily life that uses all your parts and calls you to wholeness.

The link between meditation and daily life

The link between the inner world and the outer world is your intentional effort of awareness, practised in quiet sitting and then remembered sometimes during the day when you are in action. Intentional efforts of awareness should be, at first, simple self-observation tasks. For example: 'How do I walk? Do I behave the same with each person in my day? How am I sitting right now?'

The daily effort with an inner task continues the inner work begun in quiet inner focus. It is helpful to choose specific times to explore working with an inner task, to make 'appointments' with yourself.

An inner task might be decided upon while you sit quietly in the morning. It should be written down in your journal. These tasks are like putting a stick in the spokes of a revolving wheel. They interrupt the automatic flow of endless thoughts and can remind you that you had a wish for more consciousness.

The following suggestions could help your intentional effort of awareness:

• Choose an 'earthing point' inside your body on which you keep some awareness focused. For example: your hand, the heart area.

• Keep your awareness returning to:
  – your posture
  – gestures
  – facial expressions.

• Become aware of your habitual ways of walking and perhaps try some of the walking meditations methods (see page 79).

• Work to continually 'let-go' in your body, to drop all unnecessary tension as you perform the outer work.

• Speak only those words which are necessary for the task at hand.

Such tasks have formed the 'rules' for many religious and meditative orders for centuries, although the reasons for such tasks have sometimes been forgotten. They obviously have an intent far beyond simple obedience.

The value of the inner task is not in success—since we all fail just about all the time—but in having an intent, in having some plan that will help you awaken out of inner 'sleep' and negative habits. It is also a training in maintaining precious energy. Normally you are like a sieve, filled each night with fresh energy. We gather the energy during this quiet inner focus and then leak it out during the day.

Moments of waking to self-awareness depend on preparation, practice and intent: remembering the simple task exactly, then dropping down from doing it in the mind to letting the awareness dwell in the body, in the whole of self.

There is dependence on being reminded at first—as many times as you forget! A class or a group or a spiritual director is very useful for this reminding role. Journal entries can remind you. Making a pact with a friend to remind each other and share observations can help. Since daily life often becomes familiar and routine, there is a need to consciously choose new exercises and reminding factors all the time.

Guidelines for self-study using the inner task

• Begin with quiet inner focus time each day. Then recognise a clear intention for yourself. Write the intention down in your personal journal or diary.

• Move your attention inwards to your centre before you begin any outer task.

- Agree with yourself to make this inner effort over and over, throughout the day. Willingness to begin again, as if from the start, is essential.

- Sometimes practise saying only what is necessary for the job you are doing. Experience the energy you usually use up in chatting. (This is a very revealing exercise.)

- Constantly direct your attention within. Move into divided attention as often as you remember: 50 per cent of your attention for yourself, 50 per cent for the outer task.

- Begin to make a study of the three main ways we have of reacting. Reaction is a constant—usually unconscious—activity of our psyche. We react in our mind, in our body and through our emotions. These are the types of reaction that can be observed:
  - our mind: the useless, aimless revolving chatter
  - our body: its muscular tightening and loosening, our held or shallow breath
  - our emotions: our constant likes and dislikes, our silent demands of those around us, our complaints and our self-pity.

  Observing these may save you wasting lots of reactive energy.

- Ask yourself the question from time to time: 'What are the obstacles to being present to myself right now?

- Waste no time on judgments—either self-criticism or judgments of others. This can be so draining, and produces nothing. The wish to drop judgment will reveal much. Seeing how often you judge will be a useful motivation for further inner work.

- Approach each inner effort as if it was a question. Don't say to yourself 'I will do this!' Say 'I wonder if it is possible to do this? What conditions will I need to make this possible?', etc.

When we are able to try for expanded attention the energy coming in is almost doubled—the energy of external impressions plus all the internal ones! This is a special state that has been achieved and described by serious students of many different traditional schools of inner development. Remember that divided attention is extremely difficult to achieve, so no self-criticism should be indulged in, nor should the effort be abandoned because the ego is not 'pleased' with results.

When you have prepared yourself, and remember more often, there will be moments of awakening when your perception will be more alive. These moments will include the inner effort to be connected to the sensation of the body, coming home to yourself, a new and more subtle connection to the vibration of energy. This supports non-attachment to events, so that you develop less stress in making everything turn out exactly the way you—your ego—want it. If you persevere, these moments will increase in frequency, duration and depth.

The transition moment—from your normal consciousness to a more vivid experience—can seem a bit painful. The transition moment gives a glimpse of another level of seeing the world, of being present or alive. It is similar to those special, joyous moments you may remember from early childhood when the world was vibrant and fresh. You are then not so content with a routine consciousness. If you practise this advanced work, with support, new freedom and energy enter, which make the new state much more attractive than the old hypnotic state of 'sleep'.

Can we practise expanded attention while in action in ordinary times? Am I with myself *and* the washing up? Am I with my beloved *and* loving myself? Do I watch the sunset *and* feel my own splendour inside? Can I open and focus so that the impressions coming in are increased?

Through this practice of inner watching, outer work becomes something for inner development as well. The previously strong division between inner life and outer duties can fade.

Ordinary conditions are the most difficult—cleaning the bathroom, responding to the demand of the kitchen, chatting over coffee, enduring extra long staff meetings late in December. They can also be the times in which you learn the most. If you can wake up then, there is the possibility that daily life can become a 'yoga', a way; each ordinary time has the possibility to be special.

There are several main obstacles that present themselves in almost every second of inner awareness effort: distraction, daydreaming, reaction, identification and tension. These old habits use up and drain away energy. It seems like swimming against the tide to oppose them, but can consciousness grow unconsciously? When the repressions that fuel these obstacles have been released through emotional healing work, breaking the habits, clearing the obstacles becomes a more manageable task.

To enter a moment of inner awareness, let go of everything. Drop tension, leave wandering thoughts and give up inner complaints and demands. What are you without all that? What is the true sensation then?

Before you do the housework, before you leave for your daily employment, feel again why you are doing it, reconnect with the power of your wish, remember that this day is for you—the inner and the outer! You can drop any ego about remembering or not, waste no energy on feeling a failure or a success. Waste no energy on judgment of self or others, all that is a distraction from yourself. Leave any analysis of yourself and your efforts and continue with pure observation, with opening awareness.

You may feel awkward at first, perhaps even feel a bit 'untrue'. This is because you are working against habit, stepping out of the known persona. It may also be because you are trying it with the mind. If you find that the mind is directing everything, start there, but then let the effort of awareness come from deep in the body.

Part of the cost for moving towards this new state—which opens the way to huge amounts of creativity—will be bearing a clear view of the old state: that you are rarely present, that you are almost always tense, always talking to yourself, almost always distracted from noble, positive feelings.

As this consciousness grows, you become able to feel more deeply. You become a more suitable model for the children in your care. As the organic level of this consciousness deepens, the segments of the body that contained chronic armouring relax. The energy centres, or chakras, gently awaken. The energy flows easily through its stages of expression and transformation. New ways of being emerge. New possibilities for contributing on a communal level are called from you and your creative imagination bears fruit. The wish to bring this way of being to the rising generation is strengthened.

CHAPTER TEN

Building bridges through play

... if we are willing to open our eyes to the
suffering of the child, we will soon realise
that it lies within us as adults either to turn
the newborn into monsters by the way we
treat them or let them grow up into
feeling—and therefore responsible—
human beings.

Alice Miller, *The Drama of the Gifted Child*

Improving family and group communication

This chapter looks at ways families and groups can use play to increase emotional healing and self-esteem. The games are designed to improve group or family communication. Prolonged lack of communication is a major cause of low self-esteem and emotional wounding. The exercises are less complex than most in this book.

Team-building is possible through these games. They can benefit a group of colleagues, children, parents or teachers.

In preparing for the communication games everyone in the group or family should agree to these rules:

• everyone is equal

• the dignity of each family member is respected

• no one may break anything or hurt anyone

• no one corrects another person or tells them what to think or feel

• each of you is given equal time to speak and share

• you are not trying to 'fix up' or change the other(s).

Always allow a minimum of 30 minutes for each game. Do not begin them if you have to rush off to another activity immediately after. You all need time to integrate the feelings, memories, reactions and energies that may be activated by the games.

After the games or exercises allow some quiet time for children to be still with themselves (for example, quiet activity like taking a hot bath). They need time to integrate what has happened for them in the session. This integration can be helped by:

• drawing (have paper, crayons available)

• journal writing (appropriate for older children)

• talking (be available in case they want to open up more with you after the game, but never insist that they discuss their experience).

Sometimes all of you will create drawings reflecting a new feeling of strength or inner treasure as a result of the games. Hang these drawings in a special place where they can remind you of this part of yourselves.

Once children communicate more fully and release pent-up feelings new positive and creative energy is available. This alive energy needs to be directed and this can be challenging. Have creative outlets available that will suit your child's interest, for example, drawing, dancing, playing an instrument, construction or model making, painting, writing, sport or athletic activities (that do not focus on competition).

Make an effort to really hear what children are saying about their feelings, rather than simply following the story of what they are saying. Don't immediately try to fix up or distract them from any difficult feelings.

Mirroring back is what we call deep listening to the feelings under the events or story and feeding these back. This helps children become more aware and communicate more accurately.

Mirroring children's (or each other's) feelings means that you are:

• really hearing and acknowledging them

• allowing their feelings

• valuing them and their feelings.

The need for these three things is greater than their need to feel better immediately. We can learn to trust that their feelings can resolve if given time and loving support. Our children then learn by example to hear, allow and value themselves.

General activities and exercises

Massages

Groups and families can share foot, face, scalp or back massages. There is no need to take any clothes off. Massage is particularly useful for young children at night before bed. It is often better for inviting deep, relaxed sleep than telling stories and helps children:

• feel loved and safe

• relax and sleep well

• become aware of sensations and so increase self-awareness.

Back massages can begin with you making large letters with your finger on the back. You can move on to three-letter words and simple shapes. Asking children to try to guess what the letter, word or shape is keeps their attention within their body. (See massage stories in *Emotional First-Aid For Children*, page 122.) These are some good starting points for creating spontaneous massage stories that are acted out across the back:

• One day a busy ant went searching for food …

• At the bottom of the sea lived a lively dolphin called …

• The old car was almost at the top of the hill. Would it make it? …

Dreams

Listen to each other's dreams. Dreams are a means for our unconscious to symbolically reveal inner states. Help children to record their dreams either through journal writing or drawing. Encourage children to take troubling dreams to a counsellor to be worked on. This will help them connect more deeply to and understand their inner world. This internal communication, between the unconscious and the conscious mind, increases self-awareness and prepares the way for better external communication.

It is easy to role-play the main characters or images in dreams in order to discover what they mean for the individual. (See the Gestalt role-play question sheet on page 150.)

Find more expressive activities

Families can often spend many hours in front of the television. Apart from the quality of the shows that are presented, consider the act of watching. This is a time when external stimulation is entering children's psyche. Most children need more time to express and release the burdens of the day.

Part of the normal development of children is a growing ability to cope with the stresses that come from the world around them by expressive play. Some of the exercises in this book and many of the methods of ERC actually create conditions that allow this natural release mechanism to function more effectively.

Make sure children do not watch television immediately after school. Support them to play and express. For example:

• build a sandpit and provide toys, rocks, sticks, water etc. to use in it

• encourage children to take long baths with lots of toys, dolls and containers to play with

• give them time to play or communicate before bed through drawings, colouring-in, cooking, room rearranging, listening to, playing and discussing music.

Understanding body symptoms

Underneath physical tension or pain is emotional pain. By simply placing your hand on the part of your child's body that is tense or painful, you can support them to focus and become more aware of the sensation. Encourage them to take deep breaths and talk about the pain or tension. The breath will help them to connect to the underlying emotional pain.

Ask a few simple questions of the pain to help resolution and integration. For example:

• *I am talking to the pain/tension now.*

• *Are you a deep pain/feeling, perhaps deep inside or near to the surface?*

• *How big or small are you?*

• *Do you have a colour?*

• *Do you have a shape?*

• *Are you moving or still?*

• *Did someone cause you to be there?*

• *Is there anything you would like to tell us?*

Ask children to follow with a drawing of the pain or what they felt inside themselves.

Supporting relaxation with stories

Ask children to tell you all the things that help them play, relax and have fun. Write down the list. Take turns at making up stories that include everything on the list. Is it possible to act out the story together? After the story take a moment to lie down and be still and picture all the relaxing events of the story. Then talk a little about feelings that arose in you, both from listening to the stories and from doing the activity.

Family and group communication game
Active listening

Age range: 9 years to adult.
Two, three or four members of the family or group gather in a place and at a time when you will not be interrupted.
Elect someone to read out the instructions.

1 Appoint one of the group as the time-keeper, or rotate the role of time-keeper within the group.

2 Take 5 minutes to talk about how you felt during the different activities of the day (or during the last week).

3 No one may interrupt, comment, question or add anything. You simply listen carefully to each other in silence.

4 While listening take note of the feelings mentioned. This can be done mentally or with a pen and pad.

5 When everyone has taken a turn, each of you is asked: Are these feelings over now, or still alive for you?

6 After everyone has spoken each person can take time to draw the feelings that are still current.

7 The drawings of the feelings can then be used as a basis for further discussion.

Family and group communication game
Sharing the feelings inside me

Age range: 9 years to adult.
Two, three or four members of the family or group gather in a place and at a time when you will not be interrupted.
Each person will need drawing book and crayons.
Elect someone to read out the instructions.

1 *All draw a body outline to represent yourself. (See* Emotional Release For Children, *pages 62–65.)*

2 *Lie down and close eyes and tune in to how your body is feeling. See if there are any parts inside that feel:*
   - *busy*
   - *still*
   - *angry*
   - *sad*
   - *happy.*
   Mark these on the body outlines with colours, shapes and lines.

3 *Take turns to show your drawings and talk about what you found.*

4 *Together make guesses about why the particular feelings on each person's body outline are there.*

5 *Discuss which feelings want to get out and which ones want to stay inside.*

6 *Do several drawings of the feelings that want to get out.*

Family and group communication game
Pictures on my back—sharing massage

Age range: 7 years to adult.
Two, three or four members of the group or family gather in a place and at a time when you will not be interrupted.
Elect someone to read out these instructions.

1 *Close your eyes for a moment and think up a picture of something you like very much.*

2 *Draw this picture with your finger on another person's back. You may have to do it a few times.*

3 *Ask this person to guess what the picture is and whisper the answer to you.*

4 *If they cannot guess they have to give you a brief shoulder massage. When you receive the massage say how you like it, for example, harder, softer, up a bit, down a bit.*

5 *If they do guess correctly, draw your picture on the back of the next person in the group.*

6 *Take turns to draw your picture and have one drawn on your back.*

7 *When you have finished, talk about how it felt having the picture drawn on your back and, if you had one, how it felt getting the massage.*

8 *You may want to do another round.*

Family and group communication game
Story telling to help talk about my life

Age range: 7 years to adult.
Two, three or four members of the family or group gather when and where you will not be interrupted.
Elect someone to read out the instructions.

1 *Make up and tell a story by completing these sentences:*
   - *Once upon a time, in a far-off place there lived a ...*
   - *He/she/it looked like this ...*
   - *He/she/it set out from home to search for ...*
   - *There were many dangers along the way, like ...*
   - *Unexpectedly a helper appeared. It was a ...*
   - *The most frightening thing was ...*
   - *This is what he/she/it did to become brave ...*
   - *The story ends happily with ...*

2 *Think about your story and any similarity with your life.*

3 *Discuss with the others anything in your life which is like this story.*

4 *Draw a picture from the story if you wish.*

Family and group communication game
There's an animal inside me!

Age range: 7 years to adult.
Two, three or four members of the family or group gather in a place and at a time when you will not be interrupted.
Each person will need drawing book and crayons.
Elect someone to read out the instructions.

1 *Lie down, close your eyes, stretch, wriggle, then relax and be still.*

2 *Ask your imagination to show you a picture of an amazing animal that has been secretly living deep inside you. Wait and watch in your mind's eye.*

3 *Without speaking, open your eyes and draw your animal as well as you can.*

4 *Show your drawings to each other and talk about them.*

5 *Take turns to role-play the animal. Make your body like its body, make its movements and sounds, imagine that you are the animal for a while.*

6 *Be ready to support each role-play. For example, you could say: 'Tell us about yourself, animal.'*

7 *The animal is given time to speak out a message for each family member, then for you, the person they are inside.*

8 *Each of you has a turn at being your animal.*

9 *After each role-play is finished, each of you says how it felt to hear the animal's message.*

10 *Write down, beside your drawing, the message from the animal for yourself.*

> **Family and group communication game**
> **Talking about opposites—this year, last year**
>
> Age range: 9 years to adult.
> Two, three or four members of the family or group gather in a place
> and at a time when you will not be interrupted.
> Each person will need drawing book and crayons.
> Elect someone to read out the instructions.
>
> 1 *Think about times during the last year when you felt the following*
>   *feelings:*
>   - *weak*
>   - *strong*
>   - *fearful*
>   - *brave*
>   - *lonely*
>   - *friendly*
>   - *hopeless*
>   - *hopeful.*
>
> 2 *As each feeling is mentioned do two quick drawings to represent*
>   *the feeling: one for this year, one for last year.*
>
> 3 *Use the drawings to tell the others about your feelings. Take equal*
>   *time to talk about your feelings and any memories that may have*
>   *come to you during the exercise.*

Personal development for parents

> Nothing has a stronger influence psychologically on their environment,
> and especially on their children, than the unlived life of the parents.

C. G. Jung

If parents are not already exploring some personal development work, at some stage it may be recommended that they become involved. We can only take someone to the same place we have been! Children will be able to access their feelings at a deeper level if their parents have travelled the same road. After experiencing, allowing and expressing their own emotions more fully, parents are then able to support the emotional development of their children.

Children will intuitively sense our abilities to feel and respond to their feelings. The more able we are to be undefended, the more safe children will feel to let go and be who they really are.

As your child progresses with personal development, his or her changes may call you to begin to change in some way. Children working with inner-life skills become more real and alive with their feelings. They will be more aware of their happy, sad, angry feelings and more ready and able to express themselves. This makes them more communicative and can greatly deepen their relationships.

We may have got messages while we were growing up that it wasn't okay to feel. These messages came through comments such as 'Don't be a sissy'; 'Don't cry'; 'It's not nice to be angry'; 'Be brave'; 'You are too excited, calm down'. Maybe the messages were conveyed subtly through a disapproving look. Or the feelings we had as children may have been too painful—so we shut down. As parents our children's aliveness can be a reminder of what we have closed down to in ourselves. For example, if I am uncomfortable with a child's excitement then it's probably my own excitement I am uncomfortable with and had to control as a child.

Counselling sessions may help children become aware and alive with their feelings. Inner-life skills work can be a challenge for the whole family. It can challenge them to become more open, communicative and alive. The home environment is one of the main learning places where children learn by example. If there is any discomfort in us triggered by our children, we can learn about ourselves from it.

It is quite normal for one or both parents to wish to seek ERC support during the time that their child is working with the inner-life skills or coming to counselling sessions.

Projecting parents' needs

We often project missing or denied parts of ourselves onto our children. For example, if we were never allowed to play a musical instrument we may insist that our children do. By trying to fulfil a need within us through our children we can become quite unaware of what our children truly need and want.

Through personal development work we can become more aware of ourselves and our own needs, then take steps to fulfil them. We are then better able to see our children for who they really are and what their individual needs or wants are—which may be vastly different from our own.

If there is a trait you strongly dislike in a child, you can be sure it is a trait somewhere within yourself. Usually as we grow up we learn that some of our traits earn approval and some traits attract disapproval. For example, to rest may have been judged by your parents as lazy. Rather than meet your parents' disapproval you disowned this part of yourself. You learned to 'do', 'be active', which gained approval. You live out only a part of yourself—the disowned part lies buried in your unconscious. You may project this part out onto your children and then regard them as lazy each time they rest or play.

Through inner work, you can recognise and accept these disowned parts and become more balanced and whole. This more centred inner attitude enables you to perceive your children more clearly. Maybe they weren't lazy at all, maybe they were just taking time out—as you needed to as a child.

We also project disowned positive traits onto children. Whatever we greatly admire in them is in us too—we just may not be conscious of it.

Through your own personal development you can know all of yourself and therefore let the children you are working with be all of who they are.

Most of us greatly admire young children's natural spontaneity, playfulness, joy and creativity. These qualities *are* in us too—but hidden or sabotaged. It can be difficult for us to connect with them because a lot of hurt from our past covers these qualities. Personal development work enables us to feel and release these hurts and reconnect to all of these positive qualities underneath.

If we are open to knowing ourselves, children can be our greatest teachers.

Dealing with emotional reactions to our children

There will have been a time when we were children when we didn't have our needs met as much as we would have liked or needed. There would have been hurt related to our unmet needs. If we didn't want to feel that hurt we split off from it. It's as if the feelings and memories became wiped from our consciousness and stored in the unconscious. Even though we are unaware of these feelings they very much affect our adult lives! Past unresolved feelings manifest as reactive behaviour now.

We can use our emotional reactions to our children as opportunities for our own growth and begin to:

• explore our emotional reactions triggered by our children

• connect with the feelings beneath our reactions

• discover the origin of these feelings

• release the feelings from the past which then sets us free to connect to a new positive state

• open to new ways of responding to our children.

We all have a 'hurt inner child' made up of unfelt hurts or unmet needs. It is this part of us that eventually over-reacts to our own children. It is then vital that we find the time and support to heal our own hurt inner child.

Appendices

Appendix 1:
Gestalt role-play question sheet

Children work in pairs taking it in turns to be the support person. The support person should silently read through the exercise before beginning in order to get a clear idea of it.
The support person should ask the questions slowly, giving his or her partner time to feel the answer, and then respond.

1 Say to your partner: *Relax now. You are going to pretend you are this symbol. If you are comfortable doing it, close your eyes to help you imagine you are this symbol. Now let yourself totally become the symbol. Feel your body changing, change your posture if it helps. Take some full breaths and feel how it is to be this symbol.*

2 Ask the person who is role-playing to imagine him or herself as the symbol, then answer these questions, beginning with: *I am ...*
   • *Tell me what you are.*
   • *Describe what you look like.*
   • *Feel inside, and tell me what you are made of or what is inside you.*
   • *What are your main qualities and feelings?*
   • *Tell me about your age. Are you old or young?*
   • *Do you have a particular sound or movement?* (If they do, ask them to demonstrate it.)
   • *Do you have a particular intention?*
   • *Do you have a special purpose? What are you for?*
   • *What do you want?*
   • *Do you have a message for* (person's name), *or anything you would like to say to him/her? Any advice perhaps?*

3 After a pause say: *Now slowly come back to being yourself, and then gently open your eyes. Did you hear that message? How does that feel?*

4 After some discussion say: *Now write down the message.*

5 Encourage your partner to write down the message at the end.

6 Invite them to draw the symbol, and add some words about its meaning.

7 Swap roles when you have finished or when the teacher tells you it is time to swap.

Appendix 2:
Some cross-cultural sources

The inner-life skills exercises and approaches presented in this book have been developed from the enthusiasm, study, personal experience and teaching work that has resulted from training in ERC. This new formulation of counselling and personal development approaches has been developed in Australia since 1980. ERC draws from modern consciousness research and the study of traditional systems of personal and spiritual development. It draws from Jungian, Gestalt and Transpersonal Psychology.

ERC is a dynamic experiential approach for adults, adolescents and children to support their emotional healing and self-discovery. Because of its highly experiential nature it naturally stimulates interest in new ways to expand consciousness, understand the psyche and attain a sense of well-being. Those trained in ERC experience a great openness to ancient and modern ways of exploring consciousness. The rich contributions of this book are proof of this open-mindedness.

Traditional forms of inner focus through stillness and movement

Tai Chi, Hatha Yoga, Aikido and ZaZen are ancient forms for inward focus and conscious movement that are now being more widely taught in Western cultures. Each of these traditions contributes a very practical way of experiencing increased self-awareness. Out of these respected and serious ways many different newly wrought personal growth methods are appearing.

Tai Chi was originally a Chinese martial art exercise. It incorporates a sequence of movements, performed with a meditative inner awareness, that activate a sense of well-being. Many believe the energy circuits that are enlivened by this gentle exercise positively improve physical health.

Yoga has many forms and many schools. The main forms consist of practising physical postures that stretch and relax the muscles and bring the body into optimum well-being, enabling a more subtle self-awareness. Breathing exercises, relaxation and meditation are often woven into a yoga sequence.

Aikido is a stronger Eastern martial art. Its essential practice—along with outer methods of combat—is becoming aware of the main energy centres of the body, especially the centre of gravity of the body, the belly centre, or hara.

ZaZen is a silent sitting meditation. The inward focus is returned over and over to the awareness of the inner world, allowing thoughts and emotions to fall away in time. The stillness allows inner agitation to be observed, and with perseverance and trained, compassionate guidance, a new realm of stillness and peace can be experienced.

Western personal growth pioneers

An understanding of the principles of emotional and psychological growth and healing helps us to recognise that self-awareness is a basic prerequisite for healthy development. There are many pioneering scientists and healers whose work we have drawn from in forming the exercises in this book. They have worked in the fields of medicine, psychiatry, spiritual direction, experiential self-discovery, adult education and theology.

• Dr Fritz Perls was a leader in the Gestalt movement. He not only formulated simple and effective ways of working with dream images, but emphasised the need to 'be in the moment' for healthy relating.

• Dr Carl Jung's methods for the journey towards what he called 'individuation' entailed focusing the imagination to gain access to the contents of the individual and collective unconscious.

• Drs Alexander Lowen and John Pierrakos were students and colleagues of Wilhelm Reich. They developed Bioenergetics, exercises designed to awaken the emotional and energy flows of the body and bring a greater awareness to feelings.

• F. M. Alexander researched the inter-connectedness of the way the body functioned and developed a subtle and profound technique for teaching awareness and care in the use of the body—the Alexander Technique.

• Moshe Feldenkrais developed an awareness through movement technique to harmonise the way the body and mind work together.

• Dr Ira Progoff's Intensive Journal method introduced the open-ended, self-integrating Journal Feedback techniques.

• A. H. Almaas' Diamond Approach to personal development drew from Sufism and the inner sensation exercises of G. I. Gurdjieff.

• Stanislav Grof and Christina Grof developed the technique for adults—Holotropic Breathwork—that has been used by many thousands around the world to gain first-hand experience of the transpersonal realms of consciousness. The creativity, and understanding of the psyche, of the author and contributors to this book has been greatly enhanced through the experience of breathwork.

There are many others who have inspired us and whose work we continue to adapt for educational purposes. Each has a unique gift that widens our own horizons and has a valuable contribution to the aims of the classroom, the counselling room, the retreat centre and the home.

Buddhism and Shamanism

The Eastern 'Way' of Buddhism and the modes of shamanism practised for centuries around the world have much to guide us in the search for contemporary methods of self-discovery. Although essentially atheistic, from a strictly orthodox view, they aim at creating an inner and outer balance that brings well-being and compassion for others.

While much traditional Christian contemplation focuses on the heart, on the emotional energy of devotion, Buddhism often has a focus on the energy systems of the body, especially the hara or power centre in the belly. Shamanic focus is often connected with the throat energy, which is expressed and increased through chanting, singing and sounding.

Some forms of Buddhism have a focus on teaching meditation, concentration and 'one-pointedness of mind'. Simplified versions of these exercises can help us turn within towards the source of agitation, restlessness, revolving thoughts, disturbed emotions and scattered energy. Zazen is the name of the basic silent sitting meditation. This is now widely taught in the West.

Shamanism appears in many so-called primitive cultures in South America and Asia. It is similar to many of the ancient approaches to healing and understanding nature practised across Africa. It includes methods for healing, growth, awareness, empowerment and social change. Shamanic medicine men and women were able to listen to and learn from nature and make contact with a subtle energy known as spirit. Shamanic methods of increasing awareness and empowerment include work with drums and rhythms, identification with animals and the forces of nature, and journeying into the inner world or, as they often call it, the 'underworld'.

Appendix 3:
Music

Music is a great aid to many of the exercises. Inward-turning processes can be aided by soft relaxing music that supports children into a quiet space within, without the need to use too many words. Presenters need to be ready to change music. For example, a quiet exercise may begin with silent inner focus, but this may transform into a need for some movement. After the movement sequence either quieter music or celebratory dance music could be used.

We use a drum for rhythmic work, for bringing a group together, and as a signal to begin and end small-group sharing times when children are focused on each other and not the presenter.

Here is a starting point, a few suggestions for music that we have found very supportive for particular feelings, energies and moods. Much of it is film music, as film composers are usually required to focus on one emotion or one mood. An asterisk indicates that the music is highly recommended and that children respond to it very well.

Tenderness

Geoffrey Burgon: *Brideshead Revisited* (television soundtrack, especially tracks 1, 2, 3, 4, 5, and 6)

John Barry: *Somewhere In Time* (film soundtrack, especially tracks 1, 6, 2, 8, 4, 7); the suite from the film *Indecent Proposal* (track 7)

Mark Knopfler: *Princess Bride* (film soundtrack)

James Newton Howard: *The Prince of Tides* (film soundtrack, especially tracks 2, 3, 7, 13, 22)

Ennio Morricone: *Love Affair* (film soundtrack)

Sadness, surrender

John Barry: *Out of Africa, Dances With Wolves** (film soundtracks); the compilation CD *Moviola* (especially tracks 13, 12, 6, 8, 5)

Mike Rowland: *Titania*

Stillness, relaxation, letting go, meditation

Steve Roach: *Structures from Silence*

Simon Lewis: *Southern Mystique* (especially tracks 1 and 7)

Ennio Morricone: *City of Joy* (film soundtrack, especially tracks 7, 2, 9, 15, 19, 10, 3)

Terry Oldfield: *Cascade, Illuminations*

Brian Eno & Harold Budd: *Plateaux of Mirrors*

Patrick Bernhardt: *Atlantis Angelis*

Tony O'Connor: *Bushland Dreaming, Serenity, Mariner**

Tim Wheater: *Green Dream, Before The Rains* (especially tracks 3, 4, 5, 2, 6, 1)

Jon Mark: *Alhambra*

Anugama: *Spiritual Healing**

Suppliers

For New Age and Relaxation music catalogue write to:

New World Productions PO Box 244 Red Hill Qld 4059

Appendix 4:
Four Element Sheet

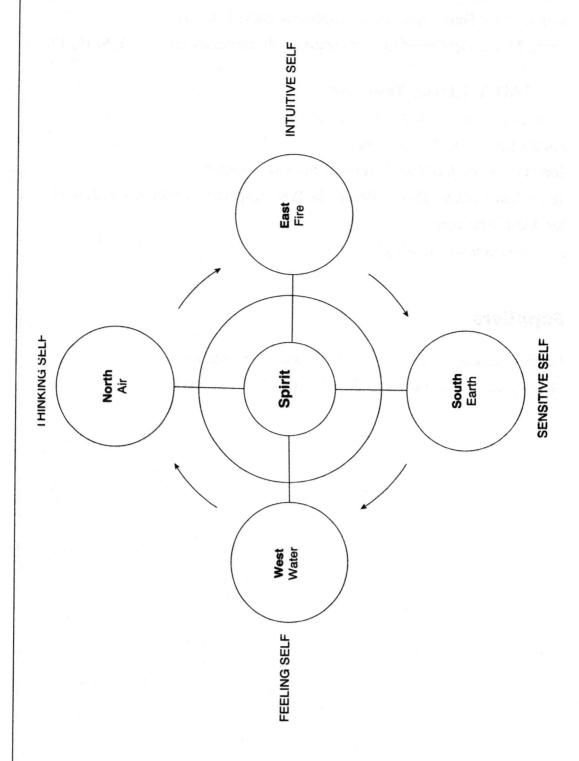

Resources

Axline, Virginia, *Dibs: in search of self: personality development in play therapy*, Penguin, UK, 1971.

Crook, Rae, *Relaxation for children*, Second Back Row Press, NSW, 1988.

Kalff, Dora, *Sandplay: a psychotherapeutic approach to the psyche*, Sigo Press, USA, 1980.

Oaklander, Violet, *Windows to our children: a Gestalt therapy approach to children and adolescents*, Centre for Gestalt Development, New York, 1988.

Pearson, Mark & Nolan, Patricia, *Emotional first-aid for children: emotional release exercises and inner-life skills*, Butterfly Books, NSW, 1991.

Pearson, Mark & Nolan, Patricia, *Emotional release for children: repairing the past, preparing the future*, ACER, Melbourne, 1995.

Rickard, Jenny, *Relaxation for children: a handbook for teachers*, ACER, Melbourne, 1994.

Resource books related to adult personal development

Bennett, J. G. et al., *The spiritual hunger of the modern child, a series of ten lectures*, Claymont Communications, USA, 1984.

Bertherat, Therese & Bernstein, Carol, *The body has its reasons: self awareness through conscious movement*, Healing Arts Press, Rochester, USA, 1989.

Durckheim, Karlfried Graf von, *Hara—The vital centre of man*, Samuel Weiser, New York, 1975.

Durckheim, Karlfried Graf von, *The Japanese cult of tranquillity*, Samuel Weiser, New York, 1974.

Feldenkrais, Moshe, *Awareness through movement: health exercises for personal growth*, Penguin Books, UK, 1980.

Gardner, Howard, *Frames of mind: Theory of multiple intelligence*, Mandarin, London, 1983.

Grof, Stanislav, *The adventure of self-discovery: dimensions of consciousness, new perspectives in psychotherapy*, State University of New York Press, USA, 1988.

Lowen, Alexander, *Bioenergetics*, Penguin Books, UK, 1984.

Lowen, Alexander & Lowen, Leslie, *The way to vibrant health: a manual of bioenergetic exercises*, Harper & Row, USA, 1977. (Note: This book is out of print, but is tremendously valuable. Look for it on friends' bookshelves, at your local library, in second-hand bookshops—it's worth it!)

Miller, Alice, *The drama of the gifted child*, Basic Books, New York, 1981.

Moore, Thomas, *Care of the Soul*, HarperCollins, New York, 1992.

Pearson, Mark, *The healing journey: a workbook for self-discovery*, Lothian Books, Melbourne, 1997.

Pearson, Mark, *From healing to awakening: an introduction to transpersonal breathwork*, Inner Work Partnership, NSW, 1991.

Perls, Fritz, *Gestalt therapy verbatim*, The Gestalt Journal, New York, 1969.

Progoff, Ira, *At a journal workshop*, Dialogue House Library, New York, 1975.

Shapiro, S. I., 'Quiet in the classroom', *Australian Journal of Transpersonal Psychology*, NSW, 1991.

Follow-up, support and on-going spiritual direction

If you wish to find contacts for support, information on workshops, training courses or individual sessions in personal development work or ERC around Australia, contact the author via the publisher, or phone him (mobile 041 9492713).

Glossary

acting out	Behaviour that is often disruptive, destructive or socially isolating, caused by reactive feelings. The actions and the causes usually do not seem to be linked.
active imagination	Intentionally giving the imagination time and encouragement to continue or complete a story, a dream, a fantasy in order to learn more about the contents of the unconscious.
active meditation	A series of actions carried out while focusing on the inner world, or preparing to turn attention within, in order to arrive at a calm and quiet emotional and physical state.
armouring	Chronic contraction of muscles that is a defence against emotions moving, expressing and being felt. For example, tightness in the chest that is holding in grief. Armouring is often only felt during still and quiet times. (See also de-armouring.)
attachment	Identification with, need for, or strong interest in something.
attention	A quality of focusing. Can be on several levels: scattered, directed, expanded or divided, or free (see pages 132–135).
awareness	A focused way of being when the person is consciously knowing what is happening in their mind, body, feelings or conscious of people and events outside themselves.
autogenic phrases	Phrases that suggest relaxation, comfort and calmness directly to the body.
bioenergetics	Specific exercises devised by Drs Alexander Lowen and John Pierrakos in the USA, that awaken and help the flow of emotions and energy within the body.
body energy	The energy sensed as flowing through the body.
body tension	The overall state of tension or relaxation as sensed in the body.
body outline drawing	A body-shaped drawing used to map feelings and sensations inside the body. Children can draw their own or use prepared outlines.
centred	A state of focused attention on the sensations in the body. Such a state enables one to become calm and more attentive, to view the world and respond from a more self-aware state.

clear	When the psyche or body is relieved of a disturbance that has been long held, there is a state of clear or free-flowing energy. A state where there are no emotional reactions or unconscious motives.
coming home	Bringing the attention back from a scattered state to focus on the body and immediate feelings and thoughts.
concentration	An activity of the mind where awareness is narrowed to focus on a specific object or subject.
consciousness	The sum of awareness from the mind, body and feelings.
de-armouring	Releasing muscular tension and allowing the flow of energy into those parts of the body that have been armoured. Bioenergetic exercises are one of the main de-armouring activities. (See also armouring.)
defences	Intended or automatic neurological, muscular, respiratory, chemical or behavioural ways of avoiding emotional pain—both internal, carried from the past—and new hurts in the present.
defended	Rejecting feedback on one's state; not wanting to know about inner life, and maintaining muscular tension in order to avoid feelings.
disowned emotion	Feelings that have been activated then denied either intentionally or unconsciously.
divided attention	Awareness focused both within ourself and outwards to the environment at the same time.
dynamic meditation	A co-ordinated series of physical exercises that aim to release agitation and bring children into a quiet, still, focused state.
earthing	The repeated effort of turning awareness within to the body which can lead to a quiet, calm state.
ego	A part of the personality which organises and controls our activity. The ego is the centre of gravity for our usual sense of identity. It also contains our defences, negative self-beliefs, and reactions to past hurts.
emotional healing	Releasing neurological, chemical and energetic patterns held in the body from past negative emotional experiences. This releases negative self-images and beliefs.
emotional pain	A way of summarising the impact of emotional neglect, hurts, disappointments.
emotional release	Allowing pent-up feelings to express through the body without restriction.

empowerment	A state of regaining a strong, positive sense of self and an attitude that one can achieve one's goals.
energy core	Describes the concentration of bioenergy that flows through the centre of the body.
energy field	Relating to the fact that human bioenergy spreads beyond the skin and can interact with another's energy.
essence	The part of our make-up that we are born with, not affected by conditioning or education. A part that cannot be wounded, but which can be covered over by moulding and negative experiences in childhood, and from which we usually disconnect.
experiential	Learning by doing and experiencing an activity.
focused creative imagination	See 'active imagination'.
Gestalt	An approach to psychological development pioneered by Dr Frederick Perls in the USA during the 1970s and 1980s. Sometimes used in this text as a shorthand way to designate the use of the Gestalt approach to reclaiming projections from symbols, images and people (see more on page 150).
hara	A Japanese term for the second chakra, or energy centre in the body located just below the navel.
higher self	The noble, positive part of the psyche that is in touch with our spiritual nature.
identifying	Merging one's identity with another, or with a belief or learned attitude.
inner child	In this text that part of the psyche that remains unhealed from childhood hurts—sometimes described as a sub-personality.
inner life	A term to summarise our combined experience of thoughts, hopes, dreams, fears, sensation, images, feelings and body states.
inner-life skills	The skills for contacting, expressing, healing and describing our inner life.
inner resources	Reserves of psychological strength, motivation, creativity and understanding, often not used in everyday life, due to overlaying self-doubts.
inner self	The often-hidden self connected to our inner life, as opposed to the persona or personality presented to the world.

integration	The act of taking time to understand, absorb, review, record or recover from new experiences.
issue	The main problem or conflict that may need to be addressed in counselling.
kinesthetic	Knowing through body awareness.
lifeforce	Strong, alive, healthy bioenergy that is rarely fully utilised, yet holds the potential for full and vital life in the body, feelings and intellectual functions.
lower self	A term—similar to 'shadow'—that relates to our often hidden, ignoble, unhealed, unresolved frustrations and reactions.
mandala	A completion drawing which results from an emotional release experience or a time of contacting the unconscious and is expressed in a circle.
mantra	A sound or word that is chanted, spoken or sung over and over to help quieten thoughts and assist inner focus.
meditation	See 'quiet inner focus'.
negative self-image	A picture of ourselves that we believe to be true—built out of criticism and non-acceptance—that has taught us that we are not capable, intelligent, creative or good enough.
non-attachment	Free and open to any outcome.
opening, to open	A state of psychological and physical expansion accompanied by an attitude of willingness to perceive something new.
outer life	The events around us and in which we participate—as opposed to the feelings, thoughts and energies inside us.
over-stressing	A way of stretching muscles that allows deeper relaxation when the stretching stops.
personal development	The on-going effort of self-understanding and adjusting outer life to be in harmony with the inner life.
personality	A learned part of us. The part that is presented to the world—sometimes like a mask. It usually covers the essence.
processing	A way of expressing the hurts in a current problem in order to discover and experience this same hurt – or reactionary energy – which really belongs to a childhood event or trauma.
project/projection	To ascribe to another a feeling that originates within oneself, but which is not conscious.

psyche	The mind, both conscious and unconscious, and its interaction with feelings, body sensation and spiritual potential.
quiet inner focus	A special time of stillness and silence where the whole attention is turned to the inner world.
resistance	Consciously or unconsciously not wanting to feel something within or open to something or someone.
role-play	To actively pretend to be something or someone in order to understand projections and reclaim projected qualities.
self-esteem	Feeling positive and confident about oneself and one's value.
spiritual autonomy	The right to one's own experience and interpretation of our spiritual nature.
spiritual growth	Increased contact with our spiritual nature that allows outer life to be directed by a higher part of the psyche.
suppression	Pushing away from consciousness unpleasant facts or feelings.
surrender	A state of deep psychological and physiological relaxation with an openness to a range of outcomes.
unconscious	The unconscious: a storehouse of feelings, memories and impulses that are not directly available to the conscious mind; to be in a state of extreme unawareness.
vision quest	In this text, means a time with nature that includes inner focus and opening to understand the symbolic meanings of nature.
visualisation	Using mental images to create pictures or stories that support states of relaxation and self-discovery.
wholeness	A sense of connection and bringing together of all parts of the psyche, accompanied by a high degree of self-acceptance.
witness	A state of presence. Watching internally, objectively noting thoughts, feelings and sensations without being distracted by them.
zazen	Quiet sitting meditation practised by Zen Buddhists.

Index of exercises

Exercises for presenters

Preparing myself to teach inner focus 21

Questions to ponder when preparing exercise 26

First questions to ponder and journal 83

Exercises that use drawing as a major method

What do my mandalas say? 31

Using colour and movement to find a gift inside 50

Exercises for 'breaking the ice'

Getting to know each other 35

Exercises for self-awareness

Humming through the middle of me 38

The sounds inside 40

Using my nose instead of my eyes 44

The ascent of the mountain 45

Looking inside myself 49

Using colour and movement to find a gift inside 50

Your dream home 52

Slow-motion for self-awareness 72

Pictures of my life on a rock 114

The well 128

Inside me/outside me 127

Visualisations for relaxation

An iceberg in the tropics 41

A fern in the forest 57

Visualising relaxation 58

Creating trust and serenity 59

The evening horizon 73

A storm at sea 112

The wild hurricane 113

Exercises for relaxation

Inviting softness 43

What is here now? 56

Exercises for self-esteem

Finding my power animal 47

A gift for now 101

The wisdom of the landscape within 103

The gift from a wise part of me 105

Feeling my strength 106

The tribal island 108

Earth people 110

My hero/my heroine 111

My reflected beauty 119

Your magic power animal 120

Inside the spaceship 122

The special message 123

Meeting your inner wisdom 124

Inside me is the very best 126

Finding my heart 129

Gestalt role-play question sheet 150

Active meditations

Basic bioenergetic exercises 64

Bioenergetic games to prepare for meditation 65

Tension and surrender 67

Earth, water, fire, air and spirit 68

Moving in slow motion 71

Slow-motion for self-awareness 72

The evening horizon *73*

Exploring the seeds of life found in darkness *74*

Relaxed walking *76*

Wandering *76*

Contact with the earth *76*

Slow-motion walking *77*

Barefoot in the park *77*

Warrior's walk *77*

I've got rhythm *78*

Zen walking *78*

Basic walking meditation *79*

Quiet meditations

Following the basic stages *85*

Guiding students towards the witness state *87*

Watching the candle flame *88*

Heart centre awareness *89*

At home in my hands *91*

Coming home *92*

Breath and energy flow through all of me *92*

The two main centres *93*

Only breath *93*

Navel gazing *94*

Return from the source *94*

Journey to the centre of the Earth *95*

Attention dissolving tension *95*

Welcoming energy pathways *96*

I live in a seven-storey building *96*

Family or group communication games

Massages *140*

Dreams *140*

Understanding body symptoms *141*

Supporting relaxation with stories *142*

Active listening *142*

Sharing feelings inside me *143*

Pictures on my back *144*

Story telling to help talk about my life *144*

There's an animal inside me! *143*

Talking about opposites—this year, last year *146*

Index

academic improvement 10
acting-out 14, 23
active listening 142
active meditation 11–12, 71–79
adolescents 16, 63, 78
affirmations 81, 117, 118
age ranges 27
agitation 18, 20
Aikido 151
Alexander, F.M. 152
Almaas, A.H. 152
anger 62
armouring 137
attention 14
attention, directed 132
attention, divided 132, 135
attention, scattered 132
attention span 12, 54
autogenic phrases 42

Bhakti Yoga 132
bioenergetic dance work 16
bioenergetics 23, 62, 64–66
body awareness 83
body imaging 62
body outline drawing 39, 143
body postures 81
body symptoms 141
bonding 10
boundary setting 28
breath 23, 63, 93, 141
breathing 38
breathing patterns 14
Buddha 22
Buddhism 152

camping 45
cathartic methods 23
celebration 29
chakras 96, 137
Christian contemplation 153
completion drawings 30
concentration 10, 25
confidentiality 28
consciousness 23
creativity 25, 99
cross-cultural sources 11

dance 23, 29
depression 62

discussions 31
disowned parts 147
divided attention 132
drawing 29, 30
drawings 101
dreams 4, 101, 140
Durckheim, K.G. von 80
dynamic meditations 15

earthing 38, 90
earthing point 134
ego 6
embarrassment 17
emotional healing 13
emotional release work 2, 15
emotional stability 10
energy centres 96
ERC principles 13
evaluation 29
expectations 22, 23, 82

fairy tales 101
families 139
family communication 139
family communication games 2
fantasies 4
fasting 45
Feldenkrais, M. 70, 152
focused creative imagination 7
four elements 68, 156

Gardner, H. 1, 2, 16, 19
Gestalt psychology 11, 151
Gestalt role-play 150
goal setting 117
goals 118
grace 61
grief 62
Grof, C. 152
Grof, S. 15, 152
group communication 139
group work 32
groups 28
Gurdjieff, G.I. 132, 133, 152

hara 26, 81, 94, 153
Hatha Yoga 132, 151
hearing 42
heart 26, 129, 153
heart centre 81, 89

hope 117
humanistic psychology 11
humming 23, 38
hurt inner child 148
hyperactivity 81

imagery 5, 17, 27, 55, 99
imagination 4, 81, 100
inner critic 18
inner focus 6, 13
inner-life skills 2, 10, 25
inner silence 24
inner task 133–134
integration 26, 29, 127
interpretation 5, 12, 30, 99

journal writing 31
Jung, C.G. 6, 12, 146, 152
Jungian psychology 11, 151

Kalff 98
karma yoga 132

leadership skills 33
Lowen, A. 61, 62, 132, 152

mandala symbolism 30
mandalas 31
mantra 26, 90
mantra prayers 23
martial art 151
massage 53, 140, 144
medicine men 153
medicine women 153
meditation 6, 20, 84
Miller, A. 138
mirroring 140
Moore, T. 130
movement 63
movement patterns 14
multiple intelligences 16
muscular holding 63
music 22, 28, 62, 145–155

negative feelings 313

Oaklander, V. 116, 117
obstacles 136
Ouspensky, P. 132

partner work 29
Perls, F. 36, 118, 152
personal development 131, 146
Pierrakos, J. 62, 152
positive qualities 13

positive thinking 117
posture 90
power animal 46, 120
prayer 24
presenter's personal development 14
presenter's preparation 83
Progoff, I. 152
projection 147
psychic phenomena 24

Qi-Gong 70
quiet meditation 12, 81
quiet sitting work 23

reaction 135, 148
relaxation 13, 25, 37, 53, 55
resistance 16, 17, 22, 28, 34
respect 8
rhythm 63
ritual 22, 24
rocking 40

sacred psychology 11
sacred texts 22
sandpit 141
sandplay 101
school programs 16
self-awareness 3, 11, 48, 82, 131
self-criticism 135
self-disclosure 33
self-esteem 5, 12, 17, 119–129
senses 42
shaking 63
Shamanism 152
Shapiro, S. I. 9
shivering 63
slow motion 70, 72
smelling 42, 44
sounding 23, 40
spiritual autonomy 8
stillness 20
stories 142
story telling 144
stress 17, 23, 62
stress management 90
surrender 7, 25, 67
symbols 29, 99, 103, 106, 114

Tai-Chi 23, 70, 151
tasting 42
team building 139
television 141
tension 18, 62, 67, 95, 141
threshold journey visualisations 100
time limits 37

touch 39, 42
transpersonal psychology 11, 151

unconscious 3
underworld 153

vibration 63
Vipassana 24
vision quest 45
visualisation 5, 41, 74, 99–100

walking meditations 75–79
wholeness 15, 99, 131
witness 15, 81, 84, 86–87
womb 15
writing 29

yoga 23, 151

ZaZen 24, 151
Zen 12
Zen walking 78